Reader's Praise

I love this book. It is a great resource for those interested in improving or achieving periodontal health.

—Stan Wint, DDS Periodontist

David speaks for thousands of compliant patients who visit dental professionals regularly. These people follow directions, use recommended products yet never reach the conclusion of their treatment plan. Is oral health beyond control? Is damage caused by insufficient care? David shines a bright light on these concerns. Read, enjoy and start to question authority!

—Ellie Phillips, DDS

David Snape saves!!! He may save teeth, money, time, and pain, but most importantly, he may save lives. Now that links have been established between the infection of chronic periodontal disease and many systemic illnesses like Diabetes, Heart Disease, Stroke and Low-weight pre-term birth his words are invaluable! Dave's new guide, "WHAT YOU SHOULD KNOW ABOUT GUM DISEASE" is a great layman's handbook about how to care for your teeth and gums. He has thoroughly researched gum disease and has written an easy to read guide for people to help themselves, yet gives balance to the need for professional care. This book is a must read for people who are afraid to go to the dentist, people in underserved areas or those who just can't afford professional dental services. Dave makes the reader aware of the signs of gum disease and what they can do to help themselves.

This book should be in dentist and doctor's office waiting areas and health clinics for the poor and working poor. He is respectful to the importance of Dentists and Hygienists in their role in helping people achieve good oral and systemic health, but also helps inform the public how to be better patients! Definitely a valuable book to have handy on everyone's bookshelf!

—Hillary Yasmer Shemin, RDH, BSDH
Marquette University Class of 1974, Holland, PA

*David Snape really gets it. Only you, the individual, can keep yourself from slipping through the many cracks in our well-meaning, but overly generic health care system. Perhaps not glamorous enough to command constant media coverage, Periodontal Disease, nonetheless has far-reaching health implications for every individual, affecting both quality of life **and** longevity.*

Drawing from his own in-depth experience and knowledge on the subject, Snape enables his reader to go easily beyond the minimal preventive care offered to most Americans. The results will empower his readers to take charge of this vital, yet often-ignored aspect of good health and wellbeing. I only wish I had this book twenty years (and several lost teeth) ago.

—John Corso, MD,
author of Stupid Reasons People Die

The book IS wonderful, and very informative! It's down to earth, in layperson language, and gives direction where one can begin searching for dental health and improving overall periodontal care.

—Dr. Tamerut Adams,
D.O. Board Certified in Internal Medicine

What You Should Know About Gum Disease

A Layman's Guide to Fighting Gum Disease

WHAT YOU SHOULD KNOW ABOUT GUM DISEASE

David Snape

Published by
Toothy Grins Publishing, LLC
12806 West 110th Terrace
Overland Park. KS. 66210

www.WhatYouShouldKnowAboutGumDisease.com

Cover/Interior design by Judi Lynn Lake

Proofing and editing by Bonnie Bachman

ISBN   978-0-9814855-0-8

Printed in the United States of America

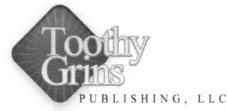

PUBLISHING, LLC

Toothy Grins Publishing, LLC
Phone 913.269.6952

12806 West 110th Terrace
Overland Park. KS. 66210

http://WhatYouShouldKnowAboutGumDisease.com

Dedication

My parents:
Thank you for being good parents and raising us well. That is no small accomplishment in today's world.

My sister, Jan:
For putting up with a thirteen-year-old brother who wasn't easy to deal with. But, you did it anyway.

My brother, Scott:
You have not been forgotten.

My nephew, Travis:
My best wishes for the brightest future.

Disclaimer

Note: Nothing in this book should be construed as medical or dental advice. Though I have made every attempt to make sure the information is correct and accurate, I cannot guarantee that it is. This is especially true when you consider that even experts have differing viewpoints. Current information and understandings might also change in the future.

This book was not intended to provide advice about gum disease or any other health condition and is for information and entertainment purposes only. You should seek diagnoses, treatment, advice, and care from a periodontist or other dental professional if you have—or think you might have—gum disease or any other oral health problem. For other health problems, visit a physician. The USFDA has not evaluated statements about the products mentioned in this book.

Additional Warning: Do not use the information, techniques, or products in this book without the expressed permission and approval of your dentist. If your dentist says no, then don't do it. Under such a scenario, you really only have two options: to follow the professional advice of your dentist, or seek the second opinion of another qualified and licensed dentist or doctor. It is very important that you do not do anything to alter or interfere with the home care treatment plan of your dentist or doctor without their expressed approval.

Contents

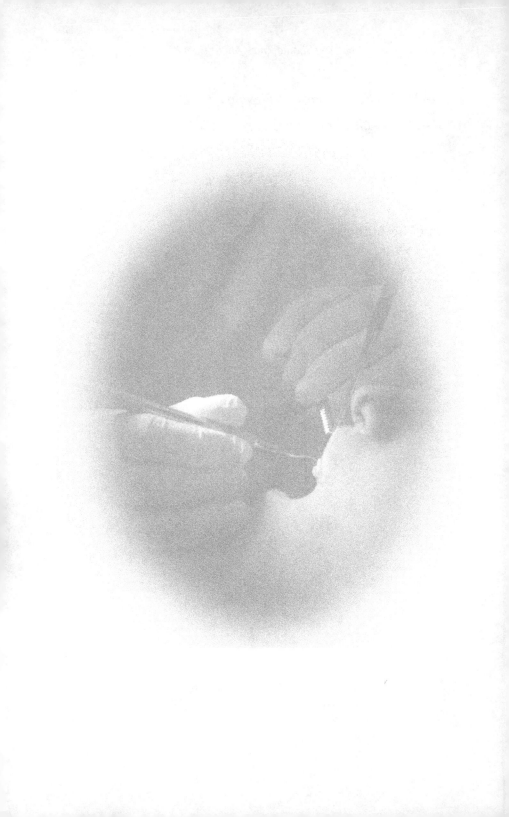

Acknowledgements

I would like to thank Jeff Olschki for donating his time to take pictures of me at Loose Park in Kansas City, Missouri for the promotion of the precursor to this book. Jeff, you are also a good listener and a solid sounding board for exploring my thoughts and ideas with. Your responses and thoughts proved to be of great benefit. Thanks especially for listening at a time when you were most needed.

Thanks to Shiling Wu for also taking photographs of me and attempting to teach me Chinese. It was great to share conversations about the nuances of the Chinese and American cultures.

I want to thank Mary Losey for her demonstration of moral character and proving to be a trustworthy friend. In a world where you expect others to let you down, it is a wonderfully refreshing experience to find good people who still value and honor the virtue of integrity. Thank you for honoring my trust. Thanks also for hours of improvisational comedy entertainment. If you were on CD or the radio, I would be a happy listener.

Thanks goes out to Susan Feder, my high school English teacher who taught me that speaking from the heart is the most powerful form of communication there is. I have not forgotten that lesson. Remembering it now brings tears to my eyes as I write this. At times when it was really important to take a stand and say or do something, that lesson proved to be valuable beyond measure. Even so, Susan, I hope you can forgive me as I still have not read Rumi.

I would also like to thank Judi Lake for sharing her insight and expertise on self-publishing. I really did not know how to finish this project and get it published. This lack of knowledge was truly slowing down my ability to continue as I began to feel bewildered by the whole process. I learned there was a lot more to publishing a book properly than you might find on the Internet or even learn directly from big publishing houses. Once I knew Judi was in my corner to guide me step-by-step, I was able to focus more on the manuscript. She took away the anxiety and uncertainty of not knowing what to do. This gave me the boost I needed to finish. You can reach Judi at her website: judilake.com.

I would like to say thank you to Dr. Ellie Phillips—a dentist who focuses on the prevention of dental disease. Having worked in a very holistic clinic in a European country, she never forgot what was possible and what can be done. Through hard work, experience, and many years of study, she has developed her own perspective on the prevention of dental disease that mainstream professionals are not likely to embrace. Thank you for taking the time to talk to me and for sharing your expertise on fighting and preventing gum disease and cavities. Your contribution to this book is most notable in your "Zellies Complete Mouth Care System," which you shared with me. Dr. Ellie has told me that her own book will be coming out in the later part of 2008. I am sure she will share her theories in detail. She has yet to inform me of the title or it would have appeared here. Dr. Ellie's website is Zellies.com.

I would like to thank the founder of the meditation practice I enjoy, called Falun Dafa. Thank you for teaching me about Truthfulness, Compassion, and Tolerance. Currently, your wonderful health enhancing practice is brutally persecuted by the Chinese government. I hope that ends soon.

If you would like to know more about the persecution and what you can do to help, visit FalunInfo.net or FOFG.org (Friends of Falun Gong). Those who wish to learn more about the incredible benefits of this powerful meditation and self-improvement practice should visit FalunDafa.org.

Thanks also to the many well-wishers who encouraged me along the way. This includes people at work as well as the other actors whom I share various stages with during this ongoing drama called life. Many people, particularly at Muddy's Coffee Shop in Kansas City, as well as folks at the Daily Dose on 135th and Quivira, would ask me about the progress of the book. These little inquiries helped me to continue when I felt like scrapping the whole project.

Thank you to all the people who contributed to this book by virtue of their conversations with me. Whether from direct conversation in person, the telephone, or email, you have helped to make this book come alive with your thoughts, ideas, experiences, suggestions, and inspirations.

Thank you again to everyone who encouraged me by simply asking how the book was coming along. You have no idea how much of a help that was. Thank you all, each and every one, thank you very much!

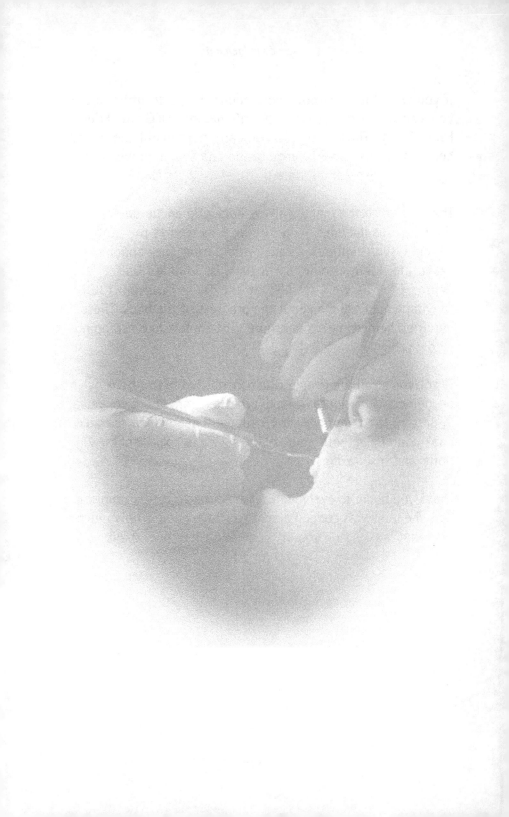

Introduction

The Day That Changed My Life

Picture this: I am sitting in my dentist's office and they tell me I have to undergo a painful and expensive process called a scaling and root planing treatment or SRP. After years of regular cleaning and treatment, they come out of the blue and drop a bombshell on me. They even wanted me to sign a document stating that it was not their fault if I lost my teeth! I told them no, and I walked out of there thinking I had just avoided a very clever scheme to get me to spend more money. I could not have been more wrong.

The hygienist had explained it would be easier to start right away with the scaling and root planing treatment rather than my regular cleaning for insurance purposes. I dislike doing anything simply because it works best for insurance. That is the same as being forced. I insisted on a regular cleaning and not the SRP.

However, there was definitely a problem that needed attention. I went home and did some research of my own on gum disease. I found out that over the years, when I was sitting in my dentist's chair with blood coming out of my gums, I was actually showing symptoms of gum disease. All that time, and all that blood, and nobody stressed how much of a problem I had! I found out that gums should not bleed at all in the dentist's office or at home while flossing. I am sure you know what my next thought was: *Houston, we have a problem.*

The hygienist had told me that I had tartar buildup under the gum line. I had to figure out a way to get rid of it so I would not have to get the SRP treatment. Again, I went out on my own and I came across a product called the Hydro Floss. I called my dentist to see if she had heard of it, and she told me not to get one. I listened to my gut instinct, and bought the Hydro Floss anyway. After five months of daily use, I amazed my dentist when I showed up without much tartar buildup along the gum line. They informed me I no longer needed the SRP treatment, and I walked out relieved. Score one for the good guys!

While I was very relieved to find out I did not need a scaling and root planing treatment, I was disillusioned by the fact that I was left to find a solution to the problem on my own.

Why couldn't they have told me about this product that could potentially save me money and, more importantly, my teeth?

Why was I paying the experts when I had to find the answers myself?

I came to the realization that many dental professionals do not focus on prevention. It is possible that prevention is less lucrative than treatment plans. It is also possible that they are ignoring advancements in the field. My dentist did not seem to know much about the Hydro Floss even though it had been written about twice in the *Journal of Clinical Periodontology*.

I saved myself time, energy, money, and pain by seeking out this information. After that ordeal, I reached an epiphany: I do not want anyone else to miss out on the answers that seem to be so elusive when it comes to gum disease. I decided to create a layman's guide to gum disease to inform others who are facing a fate similar to my own. Along the way, I have experimented with a plethora of techniques and products. Some worked for me, and some did not. I will tell you what works for me in the hopes this information will prove to be useful to you.

I have seen a good amount of fakes out there. There are people who claim to be experts on things, and later you find out that all they have is an uncanny ability to wing it. What is even more misleading is that they make it sound official! They fill your head with pipe dreams about guaranteed results and magic cures. They actually make you believe that if you listen to them, your life will change for the better. I need to put something out front right away: I am not one of those guys.

I am also not a dentist nor a doctor. I do not pretend for a second to have those credentials. I am a dental patient and a layperson; an average guy who just happened to have gum disease as many other people do whether they know it or not. I am an expert only on my own personal experience. It is my hope that by sharing my experience, I may possibly help someone else.

Inside this book, you will find more than a couple of stories about my encounters with dentists and other dental professionals over the years. Some are good, as in the case of my current periodontist. Some are not good. Please understand that I am not trying to harm the dental profession or tarnish its reputation with the negative stories.

If you are a non-dental professional, as I am, this book was written primarily for you. I experienced my own frustration at not understanding gum disease. Not knowing what to do can be the source of great anxiety. I know. If this book can cut through the mystery, misconceptions, and angst about gum disease, then I feel it will have fulfilled part of its purpose.

Much like a biography or a set of memoirs, my aim is to recount a period of my life. I talk about fighting gum disease in this book, and I talk about preventing it. I never talk about diagnosing it, treating it, or curing it. Those things are what your dentist is for. I will tell you how I fought—and continue to fight gum disease, as well as the tools that I have used and found to be useful in that fight. I do not intend to give you advice. If you want advice, diagnosis, or treatment, then you should visit your dentist or periodontist. In fact, if you are not already under the care of a dentist, then you should put this book down and make a few phone calls. This is very important. Being under professional care is critical to your health and to the health of your gums.

There are many reasons I bring this up. I am pretty sure that some readers have not visited a dentist or periodontist for some time. If that is the case, you really should go—and do not stop going ever again. The stakes are pretty high, and you should not risk the consequences. It is a coin-toss that you could lose every time.

Whether or not you have gum disease, you should definitely be under the care of a dentist or periodontist. In the case of other non-dental health problems—or suspected health problems, you should be a under a physician's care.

A case in point: The other night I received a call from a woman who told me neither she nor her husband had been to a dentist for a while. The husband finally got a job with decent health care benefits. When he went to the periodontist, he found out that he needed some pretty drastic treatment to save his teeth. Four of his front teeth needed some type of metal brace to keep them from falling out. It sounded like he needed a lot of surgery to fix the problems he had developed over the years. Even with his benefits and insurance, he was going to have to pay a pretty hefty sum of money to rectify his problem.

As you might already be aware, as many as eighty percent of adults suffer from some form of gum disease. In most cases, this does not have to be. A good number of people, as in my personal example, are not even aware they are suffering from gum disease. This could be part of the reason that the Surgeon General labeled dental disease a "silent epidemic."

The sad truth is that even if you did everything I have done to fight back against gum disease, it might not work for you. You might not get the results that I have, and you might not be able to effectively stop or prevent gum disease. Even in medicine, there are no guarantees. Results vary based on a number of factors. Medicine is not a science; it is an art. You can take a specified quantity of a certain drug and insert it into two human bodies in correctly specified doses, and get two entirely different results. In other words, you cannot take a known quantity or quality and add it to an unknown quality or quantity and get exactly predictable results. One plus X does not equal 2, unless X equals 1. Since, as in the case of different human bodies, we do not know what X equals, the answer to the equation cannot be predicted accurately every time. Oftentimes, there is nothing more than an educated guess guiding you. Has your doctor ever had you "try" one medicine only to discover that another works better, or has fewer side effects? See what I mean?

Another thing you should be aware of is that fighting gum disease is a lifetime daily process. Unless current technology improves, you will not be able to stop fighting gum disease any time soon. Therefore, I do not claim to be free of gum disease.

Stopping it in the first place and preventing it from coming back will be a lifetime battle. You should realize that this is what you are facing. In fact, you have already been facing it.

Did you know that the harmful bacteria that can harm your gum tissue will start to grow within just a few hours after plaque has formed? Unless the plaque that provides the environment for these bacteria to multiply is removed daily, you will most likely see gum disease develop at some point. There is a very rare two percent of people who will never develop gum disease, even under such conditions. However, chances are pretty high that you are not in that group, as I am not.

Therefore, I want you to understand that there are no quick solutions or easy answers to free you from the responsibility of the daily fight against gum disease forever. Such easy answers do not really exist. Magic bullets are what myths are made of.

My simple background in the life sciences did not tell me much or prepare me for the onslaught of gum disease. Knowing this to be the case, it is easy to see how bewildering it could be to someone without such a background. I was ignorant enough to believe it was normal for my gums to bleed during a professional dental cleaning. Unfortunately, the professionals working on my teeth during those years never impressed upon me what that bleeding signified—that is, until they were ready to administer a costly treatment.

It was an interesting journey from being clueless to understanding the "big picture." My wish is that this book will give the layperson a similar understanding and save him or her from the kind of anguish and heartache that goes along with being in the dark about something as important as what is going on within your own body.

Home care is an absolute necessity, and professional care is equally important. You are not likely to win the battle against gum disease by ignoring either one. A professional can help you in ways that you are probably not aware of. However, virtually every dental professional out there will tell you that every patient must do a good job of home care on their own, as well. Both are needed. That is universally agreed upon.

If you find this information to be of value, consider telling others. If you are a dentist or periodontist, consider keeping this book in your office—or even giving each patient a copy as a gift when they come for their initial or follow-up exams. They will remember you for it. As you are undoubtedly aware from your experience and education, gum disease is a serious epidemic and people, in general, really have little to no idea of what is going on. They really should have a working understanding that can serve them well.

Knowledge is potential power, and I believe we should all strive to empower others as best we can. This is my little contribution towards that end. I invite you to join me by spreading the word about information on gum disease. Let us make sure everyone at least has the opportunity to understand what gum disease is and how it can be prevented or defeated.

From this book, the everyday person can gain an understanding of what can happen and what to look out for. They can also get a feel for what questions to ask, and when it is appropriate to seek a second—or even third opinion. Each person should also become more active in his or her own situation and understand better what patients' rights are.

There are borderline unethical practitioners in every profession. Unfortunately, I have had some questionable experiences with practitioners in the dental health field. If you are a dental care professional, I am quite certain you have witnessed or experienced something sometime that seemed questionable to you as well.

The best course of action for both patients and doctors is to not hide these things or even downplay them. It is important for these stories and informative examples to be out in the open. Though you could disagree with me, my opinion is that patients should not go to a dental practitioner completely ignorant and be blindly obedient to anything the practitioner does or says. Instead, I believe patients should take an active role in their care. They should learn what questions to ask and what kind of answers they should expect.

In this way, average people can begin to learn about superior home care. They can begin to understand the whole process of gum disease and become active in restoring and maintaining the health of their gums so that their teeth can serve them for a life-time. Also, they can be spared from the contribution gum disease makes to other diseases, such as heart attack and stroke, as well as pre-term and low birth weight babies.

I have additional experiences with several dental practitioners that reflect poorly both on their character and their ethics. Again, please understand that this is not about the profession, only my experiences with a few practitioners over the years. Drilling a reversible pulpitis does not count as preventive dentistry, as one dentist tried to tell me.

I am not the only one with a few horror stories to share. I have talked to many people over the years and have heard some of their negative experiences as well. On more than one occasion, I have been told stories of how one doctor told a patient she had

X amount of cavities. When she went to another dentist, no cavities were found.

Some professionals are tempted to take liberties they should not take. Many patients are too ignorant about matters relating to oral health to know when their interests are not being best served. Some doctors could label these as gray areas. I do not often see them this way. Stories like the ones above bother me at a deep level.

I suspect that any dental professional who reads this—if they honestly reflect on their own experiences and knowledge of the field—will have to acknowledge there are some problems they have also noticed among dental professionals. This applies as well to a lack of serious effort on a national or even global scale to educate the layperson about gum disease and how to prevent it, much less how to fight an existing case.

There are many ethically sound dentists who do not enter those gray areas and do not take advantage of patients' ignorance of matters relating to their oral health. They maintain high moral and ethical standards and expect the same of their colleagues. In addition, they genuinely care about their patients and want the best for them. Those are exactly the professionals I want to partner with to spread the word about gum disease.

To Dental Professionals
If you are a dental professional, I extend an offer to partner together with you to help laypeople everywhere have a better understanding of what gum disease is and how it can be defeated or prevented in the first place. If it cannot be prevented, then let us work together to help people understand what they can do

to fight against it. Gum disease is a serious epidemic and people, in general, really have little to no idea of what is going on.

The average person just needs to know a few details and tidbits of information that he or she currently lacks. Keep in mind that repetition is the key to learning. Having better educated patients would make things easier on you, as well. It would relieve a lot of anxiety, and help to eliminate the barriers that block people from seeking treatment in the first place. Understanding the reasons behind your recommendations would help insure compliance too.

You can play a major role in helping your patients learn how to fight and prevent gum disease. It would be useful to take advantage of every opportunity to educate your patients and to do so tirelessly. It is a service that will have far reaching and beneficial implications for people's dental health as well as your own practice. This would also benefit society at large as the base level of understanding would be raised amongst the population. You will be ultimately helping to raise the quality of life for people everywhere. Each visit to your office is a prime chance to teach patients what they should know.

Wouldn't it be great if all your patients understood why you need to scrape and scale their teeth so diligently? Wouldn't it be so much easier to work with them if they had an appreciation of the need for professional cleanings? You will be so much more successful when they understand how much you are really helping them. Then, perhaps there would be less people stating that they hate to visit the dentist.

Together, we can see to it that the average person has a greater understanding of dental health and what they can do to prevent gum disease.

To The Layman

I have digressed too far now. This book is for average people, non-professionals, people just like me. Readers must remember that professional care is first and foremost. At the same time, having excellent home care skills will help you fight or prevent gum disease. Both professional care and home care are important for you to be successful in eliminating gum disease or stopping it from appearing in the first place. Be sure to work closely with your care provider of choice.

Chapter 3 is focused on home care. I have included many of the useful tools, products, and techniques I have discovered along the way.

Do not take this book as a substitute for professional care, because it is not meant to be one. If you are not happy with the advice of any one dental practitioner, you have every right (and are encouraged) to seek the second or even third opinion of others. In any case, make sure you are under the care of a dental professional.

I do hope this book will provide you with information about gum disease and fighting it that you did not previously have. I am pretty sure that it will. Keep in mind that knowledge is power, but only when it is put into use. Once you "get it," taking action will be the pivotal key to your success.

Warm Regards,
David Snape
Author: *What You Should Know about Gum Disease*

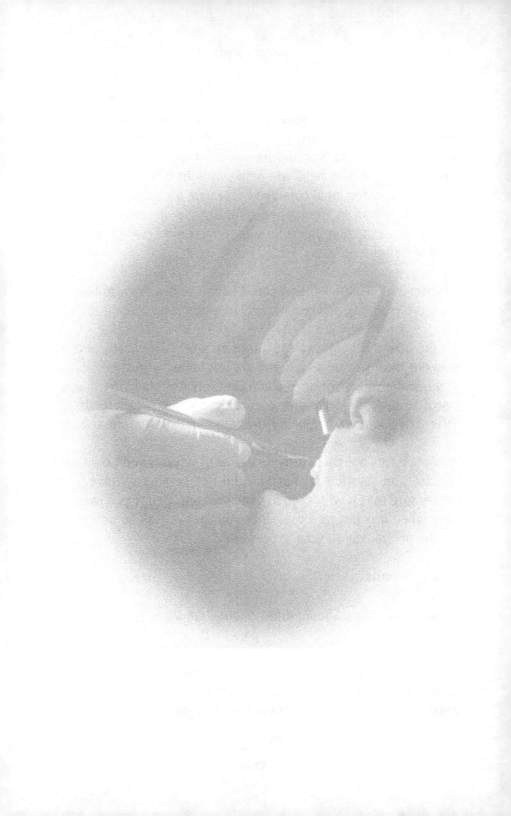

Better to be wise
by the misfortunes of others
than by your own. —Aesop

Discovering An Unwanted Guest: Gum Disease

Surprised By Gum Disease

IMAGINE THAT YOU have just arrived at your dentist's office for what you thought would be a routine dental cleaning and examination. Instead, your dentist tells you that you need a scaling and root planing procedure performed. You are told that you need this because you have mild to moderate periodontal disease. Calculus, also known as tartar, has built up under your gum line and must be removed. If something is not done, you could be in danger of losing your teeth. They want to start right now, today! What do you do?

You think: I have always been diligent about brushing and flossing. You then begin to wonder:

> *How did this happen? What about my last five visits to this office? Why do I suddenly need this procedure? What kind of expense and trauma do I need to endure now? Why do they want to start today?*

This was my experience and the source of much pain and frustration. The ensuing quest to understand and conquer gum disease provided the impetus for the creation of this book. Along the way, I learned that gum disease is a big problem for more people than I ever imagined. Some know they have it while others are not even aware of it—yet.

Finding out that you have gum disease can be quite a shock, especially when you have gone through your life taking scrupulously good care of your teeth and gums. You are not alone as up to eighty percent of adult Americans have some form of gum disease. That is likely to hold true for the rest of the world as well.

Scaling and root planing is a relatively intensive, under-the-gum (subgingival) cleaning. It could be painful to the point that you will need to be given an anaesthetic to numb your nerve endings as the root surface is scraped down to remove the built up calculus. Sometimes the anesthetic is not needed, but often it is. This hardened substance has to be eliminated; it harbors the bacteria responsible for your condition.

Noticeable effects from gum disease do not happen overnight. It very often takes years to progress to a point where you become aware of gum recession or the teeth become loose. Gum disease can be fought—and the battle won, but why not prevent it in the first place? Once the damage is done it is very hard to reverse.

The percentage of people suffering from gum disease seems really high, and this could mean that regular brushing and flossing is not enough to prevent it in many people. Unfortunately, by the time someone realizes they have gum disease, the damage has usually already been done. If you pay close attention, I am sure you will notice that someone you know is exhibiting signs of gum disease.

Gum recession—growing "long in the tooth," developing a toothy grin—these are euphemisms for the visual damage of gum disease. Yet these are merely the cosmetic effects. Gum disease can also cause a person to lose teeth. No matter how expensive or expertly designed, no denture or implant is a perfect replacement for your natural teeth.

Can gum disease be a precursor or contributor to more serious conditions such as heart disease, stroke, lung infections, and premature and low birth-weight babies? The continuing research shows there does appear to be some correlation. The official jury is still out, but more professionals are accepting the likelihood that there is a real connection. Many theorize that during an active case of gum disease there is a constant influx of bacteria into your bloodstream.

What is gum disease? How can you prevent gum disease? How can you stop it from progressing any further if you already have it? Let's take a look.

Signs of Gum Disease

Like many people, I had a small amount of bleeding when brushing or flossing my teeth. At the time I did not think it was a big deal, but it was a signal that I had gum disease. Bleeding by itself is not a conclusive indicator of gum disease, but bleeding gums can also indicate various kinds of other diseases, health conditions, or even reactions to medicine. If your gums bleed or are sore and tender when you floss, you most likely have a problem with gum disease. A diagnosis from your dentist will be needed to be certain and to rule out other possibilities.

I experienced even more bleeding during my regular hygienic cleanings at the dentist's office. In fact, the hygienist would

have a pile of blood tainted gauze when she was finished cleaning my teeth.

Like most people, I did not realize that it is *not normal* to bleed a
little while brushing, flossing, or during regular dental cleanings.
Yet, a person can still have gum disease even if there is no bleeding
during these activities.

Some of the other indicators of gum disease are:
Persistent bad breath
Red, swollen, or tender gums
Painful chewing
Loose teeth
Sensitive teeth
Gums pulling away from the teeth
Teeth that have shifted in position
Pus anywhere around your gum line

This is not an exhaustive list; there could be other similar symptoms, as well. Please do not think you are home free if you do not
exhibit any of these symptoms; they are not always evident until
the disease has progressed. By the same token, try not to be
frightened if you have just one of these symptoms in isolation.
They can be caused by other factors and are not conclusive. They
are merely indicators and still require the diagnosis of a dentist or
periodontist. However, some of these symptoms could indicate the
existence of even more severe diseases. If you have any of them,
please make an appointment with your dentist or periodontist
immediately. Self-diagnosis can get you into trouble. You need a
trained professional to verify if you have—or do not have—gum
disease. The untrained who think they know the difference are
frequently wrong.

What is a Periodontist?

There is a specialization within dentistry called periodontics. This specialization focuses on gum health and disease treatment. Periodontists have specialized training, knowledge, and experience in gum health and disease and are perhaps the most qualified to care for your gums. They can provide the maximum help and insight into your condition. Visit your dentist when you have a cavity or other problem relating to your teeth. Visit your periodontist for any problems or suspected issues with your gum health. It should be noted that both dentists and periodontists have training in regards to gum disease. Both are considered qualified to treat gum disease, but the periodontist has more training, and gum disease is often the focus of his practice.

You would want to visit a cardiologist rather than a general medical practitioner when you know you have a problem with your heart. Obviously, the cardiologist is going to provide a higher degree of care on matters relating to the heart muscle and its health. He is going to be more on the cutting edge compared to a GP (general practitioner). Plus, it is more likely that he will be aware of the latest developments. His experience with the heart is going to exceed the GP. The same idea applies to periodontists in matters relating to your gum health.

I have experienced care from both general dentists and periodontists. My experience is that the periodontist was able to help me to a much greater extent than the general practitioner. He also saw and told me about many things that the general dentist did not. He was able to find a problem that the general dentist either missed or neglected to warn me about; I had a "subgingival" defect which is something my dentist never told me about. There was actually a study done that affirmed general dentists are not always focused on the detection and prevention of gum disease (NTIS order # PB81-221780 – Page 12).

There is no need to wait for a referral, either. My dentist never suggested that I go to a periodontist. I decided to go on my own. It was definitely worth the visit. Sometimes you have to utilize a stronger grip on the reigns of your personal health care. Unfortunately, even professionals are not always thinking in terms of what is best for you.

Sometimes the "standard of care" works against the best interest of the patient. I believe that our current system of health care in the United States sometimes impedes dental professionals from doing what is best for the patient. The system often forces them to work under the overarching concern of what insurance will pay for.

The difficult part for many people is actually going to the dentist. Understandably, we fear pain, bad news, expense, and more pain. This fear factor needs to be overcome. Your gum health and your ability to keep your teeth for the long haul hang in the balance. An ostrich will bury his head in the sand to avoid trouble. Similarly, in the case of your dental health, ignoring the problem will not make it go away. I recently spoke to a man who spent twenty-one thousand dollars to get his teeth fixed. *What is that saying? An ounce of prevention is worth a pound of cure.*

In order to diagnose you, the dentist or doctor must see you in person, take a medical history, examine your mouth closely, take x-rays, and possibly administer or order other diagnostic tests. Diagnosis is both an art and a science, and there are many intertwined factors that must be taken into consideration. It is impossible to do a remote diagnosis, so there is no way around it—you must see a doctor or dentist in person. Attempts to self diagnose could lead to disaster. The human body is too intricate for the layman to attempt self-diagnosis. The consequences of such behavior could be heavy.

A concerned woman wrote to me that she actually had blood in her mouth every morning when she woke up! Needless to say, she was very worried. I advised her to visit her dentist immediately, but she said she could not afford to go. In actuality, she could not afford the risk of *not* going. With gum disease, the bleeding is not usually that severe. Even minor bleeding warrants a visit to a periodontist, let alone a severe situation such as hers. Having lost touch after a few brief conversations, I do not know what happened to her. I sincerely hope that she went to a periodontist for diagnosis and treatment.

Contributing, or "Risk" Factors for Gum Disease

Gum disease is caused by anaerobic bacteria that grow under a biofilm called plaque. Plaque is the enemy when it comes to gum disease: it can become tartar, or calculus. I will elaborate on plaque and how we can fight against it a little more later on. For now, I am going to talk about some factors that could contribute to the start or continuation of gum disease. These contributing factors are not in any particular order.

Genetics: What we inherit from our biological parents is a factor. Some people are very fortunate, because they are not likely to develop gum disease even when they do not do much to care for their oral health. I call them the lucky ones because they account for only about two percent of the adult population. On the other side of the spectrum, you have another two percent who are likely to develop gum disease no matter what they do. The rest of us are in the other ninety-six percent. We have to work—to varying degrees—in order to be successful at preventing or checking the progression of gum disease. There are a number of factors that can affect how much work is needed; genetics is just one of them.

Hormones and Pregnancy: Hormones and pregnancy are both factors that elevate a woman's risk for gum disease. You have possibly heard of "pregnancy gingivitis." That little guy or gal growing inside of you uses up quite a bit of your body's resources. I do not believe anyone has conclusively pinpointed the exact reason why pregnancy or hormonal changes cause an increased risk for gum disease. However, they both have been found to do so. Also, there was a study done in 2005 concluding that pregnant women with gingivitis are at a higher risk for giving birth to a premature baby or a baby with low birth weight (PMID: 16277587). It takes time for new information to be assimilated into the mainstream. Therefore, all professionals might not agree with this information. However, this knowledge is becoming more widely accepted with each passing day.

Smoking: It seems like there are plenty of good reasons to give up smoking. Here is yet another. Smoking is a contributing factor to the development of gum disease. This could be because of the smoke's effect on the immune system or the direct effect of the smoke on gum tissue. Smoking dries out the mucous and saliva-producing tissues of the mouth, and smoke is also toxic in nature. Any of these reasons—and more—can be why smoking contributes to the progression of gum disease. It makes sense, right? Smoke is poison and poison harms the tissues of the body.

Allow me to digress. When I took gross anatomy, our team's cadaver was that of a man who had smoked for many years. Guess what we could smell when we opened the chest cavity? The odor of cigarette smoke hit my nose and was quite revolting. Keep in mind that cadavers are soaked in formaldehyde for many months before they make it to a gross anatomy lab. You would think that would have made a difference but it did not. You can smell smoke when opening the chest cavity of a former smoker despite the cadaver's lengthy soak in formaldehyde.

There was something even more striking about our cadaver. The lungs were black inside and out. If you sliced the lung in half, it was the same degree of blackness on the outside as the inside all the way to the very center. When I say black, I mean coal black. Non-smokers' lungs, by contrast, are usually pink.

I threw in this tidbit to entice you to quit smoking, if you have not yet done so. If you have never smoked, pat yourself on the back for a job well done.

I have put together two resource pages to help with quitting smoking:

> 1. http://tobeinformed.com/quitsmoking—This page contains links to products for self hypnosis as well as government-sponsored pages and other resource pages for quitting the smoking habit.

> 2. http://tobeinformed.com/282—This page provides links to natural methods for quitting smoking. One is an herbal supplement. Another is through the use of magnets. Both are very interesting options to help quit smoking and perhaps avoid some of the painful side effects of quitting.

Chewing tobacco creates similar problems to smoking and could actually be worse as the chew rests against your gum tissue for extended periods of time. The chew is toxic to the body's tissues and the chemicals are harsh and damaging.

Diabetes: One challenge associated with diabetes is that it increases your risk for gum disease because diabetes increases your risk for infection. Gum disease is essentially a bacterial infection of your gum tissue and supporting structures.

David Snape

Stress: Everyone has heard that stress decreases the ability of your immune system to fight off invaders. Therefore, stress also raises the risk of developing gingivitis or gum disease. When the immune system is compromised, the bacteria constituting an infection have a better chance to grow. When you are stressed and worried, you help create an optimal environment for bacteria to thrive in.

Medications: Some medication can contribute to the development of gum disease. As you will see in the question and answer chapter of this book, some antidepressants can cause the mouth to dry out. A dryer environment is good for the bacteria to grow more rapidly. Your saliva suppresses that growth. Sleeping with your mouth open or mouth breathing can have a similar effect.

Important Note on Medications: It is always a good idea to read the side effects of medications you are taking. Unfortunately, they will not say something like, "this medication might contribute to the beginning or progression of gum disease." Instead, they will merely list "dry mouth" as one of the potential side effects. When it comes to medications, the general information is there, but it is up to you to connect the dots. Fortunately, you do have a professional resource at your disposal. There is a licensed pharmacist attached to the place where you pick up your medication(s). Ask the pharmacist to review the side effects with you. If your primary concern is gum disease, then ask specifically about what might cause a reduction in saliva production or how the medication could affect your gum tissue. You can often have the pharmacist print out a list of side effects for you. Simply ask. You might also ask if the medication has any side effects that cause any other problems relating to gum tissue and its health.

Other Disease and Treatments: Illnesses like AIDS or treatments for cancer can wreak havoc on the body, and particularly the immune system. Obviously, this can make you more susceptible to additional diseases, including gum disease.

For a list of HIV resources: http://www.tobeinformed.com/hiv

Confirmation of Gum Disease

There are two primary tools and techniques the dentist or doctor uses for confirming the existence and extent of gum disease: diagnostic x-rays and periodontal probing. X-rays can show a number of problems including the loss of bone. Periodontal probing is when the practitioner measures the extent of pocket depth. Pocket depth is the depth of the unattached tissue around the tooth. Anything beyond 3 mm (millimeters) is considered to be a problem. A record will be made of your readings. Your dentist or periodontist will use these and other factors to contribute towards his or her final diagnosis.

Pay special attention to your pocket depths. This will be an important gauge to measure your progress in the future. On an initial periodontal exam, all the gum tissue should be measured on both the lip side and the tongue side of your teeth. This record should be used as a baseline and will show your improvement over time. You want to make sure your hygienist always informs you of any pocket depth over 3 mm. By comparing the results to your baseline, you can keep your finger on the pulse of your gum health. Of course, this information can be used to see if the gum health has declined as well. If you develop additional pockets between visits, then you should consider refining your home care procedures. In fact, if you are not seeing a decrease in pockets altogether, then you probably need to fine tune things at home. We will discuss home care tools and their uses in Chapter 3.

If your hygienist does not automatically tell you what your pocket depths are, ask her to do so. Ask that she point out the exact areas that are greater than 3 mm. Do this on every visit. This will help you to identify your trouble spots—areas that you will want to pay special attention to during your home care. Insist on having these spots pointed out, if necessary. This is crucial to understanding where you must do the most work in your home care.

It never hurts to study up a little on matters relating to your health. You will learn a lot and possibly be healthier in the long run. My personal philosophy is to learn all I can so that I possess a semi-qualified opinion when evaluating the advice provided to me by professionals. I do not like blindly following advice, even from professionals. Being informed also helps me to understand all the reasons "why" in order to be more compliant with the doctor's recommended treatment plan. You are more likely to follow through if you understand why you must do something.

In this book, you will discover that when it comes to health issues, you should be working under the guidance of your doctor. Specifically, in the case of gum disease, working with your dentist or periodontist as well as developing excellent home care habits is essential to preventing or stopping the progression of gum disease. These are the two major aspects of winning the battle for your periodontal health. Relying on one alone can spell failure.

Some of us have to work harder at home care than others for our gums to remain healthy. Genetics, smoking, general health, stress, bacteria, and many other factors contribute to whether you will have a relatively easier or harder time caring for your gums. It is not fair to the individual who has to work harder, but that is how it goes.

What Is Gum Disease?

The term "gum disease" is synonymous with the term "periodontal disease" and is actually an umbrella term referring to a number of different stages of the same disease. I shall avoid going into a detailed description of all the various stages; it is all gum disease and we want to prevent and eradicate it all the same.

Gingivitis is the mild form of gum disease, and is characterized by red, puffy, and swollen gums. Basically, the gums are inflamed due to the presence of the toxins that bacteria are secreting. Left unattended, the condition usually progresses into worse classifications of gum disease.

If you have been told you have gingivitis, you must take action to stop it as soon as possible. Though the damage from gingivitis can be reversed, who is to say exactly when you will slip over the line to more progressive stages of gum disease? Will someone be there to tell you the exact moment that happens? Probably not. Take a diagnosis of mild gingivitis very seriously. You must take action immediately to prevent the progression of gum disease and receding gums.

There are many thousands of kinds of bacteria that can make a home in your mouth. Even the experts are not completely sure how many different kinds of bacteria there are. It is like the Amazon Rainforest—new species are often found there that were never known to exist before. In addition, even experts in microbiology have not distinguished between which of those thousands cause gum disease and which do not. They know some that do, but it is assumed that there are other varieties that do, too. The work of cataloging all of those different types is not nearly done yet.

You will see the term "anaerobic bacteria" come up next. Let me briefly explain it. There is no mystery here and the concept is pretty straightforward. Anaerobic is a descriptive term for bacteria that produce energy under conditions of not having oxygen present. The cells in our own bodies can do this, too, but they are not very efficient about it; it is a short-term measure at best. Bacteria can do it on a regular basis, however.

The toxins that anaerobic bacteria secrete as waste products under and around the gum tissue cause gum disease. Though perhaps a little graphic, these bacteria use our mouths as a bathroom, filling areas around the gum line and onto the teeth with their waste. These waste products, which are acidic, cause both gum disease and cavities. They are toxins that damage our tissues. These anaerobic bacteria flourish under a thin biofilm called dental plaque. *This also hints at the secret to defeating gum disease.*

The biofilm is easy to disrupt. However, you have to do it every day without fail. Consistency is the key. There is no need to be hard on your gums, but there is a need to take care of them consistently, day in and day out. When the biofilm remains intact for too long the anaerobic bacteria begin to flourish. Therefore, you want to remove the plaque daily to avoid the proliferation of anaerobes (anaerobic bacteria). The dental plaque that has not been removed for a period of time allows the excessive growth of anaerobic bacteria. More acid secreting bacteria means even more toxins dumped into our mouths. All dental professionals advocate the daily removal of plaque.

How long is that period of time? In other words, how long does it take for the bacteria to have enough cover from oxygen, underneath the biofilm, to start using anaerobic means of producing energy and begin to secrete the waste products that can cause tooth decay and gum disease? I am not sure anyone has a good answer for this question. It could happen in as little as a few hours, depending on the situation and the conditions in your mouth. Researchers do know that the biofilm begins to reform virtually immediately after being disrupted. The beginnings of biofilm formation can be detected in as little as thirty minutes after disruption.

The problem here is that when you eat, the anaerobic bacteria already in your mouth will start processing the meal you just gave them into acid waste products. This is why you will hear some people say to brush and floss after snacks and meals.

It is important to be proactive and to attack and disrupt the plaque before the anaerobes have an opportunity to thrive. Continual removal of plaque is key to your gum health. The more plaque that harbors bad bacteria, the worse your problems with cavities and gum disease can become. You must work to remove this hazard called plaque as diligently as your personal situation requires.

I just said the biofilm is easy to disrupt, but do not get too excited. There is another aspect to this problem. You might not be able to reach every spot on your teeth and near your gums each time you do home care in order to prevent the anaerobes from proliferating. Herein lies one of the pitfalls. If you miss one area, you have a problem. If you consistently miss any area, you have an even bigger problem. This is also one more of many reasons why you need professional care. You need someone else to make sure you are getting everything, and to point out the spots you could be routinely missing.

Despite this, you must not underestimate the power of daily plaque removal. It is the key to defeating or preventing gum disease. You cannot give up, just because it is hard to get everything. Perhaps some of the methods spoken of in Chapter 3 will help fill in some of the gaps that general brushing and flossing can leave behind.

If plaque and the anaerobic bacteria that live in plaque are the cause of gum disease, then you now know two things: One is what causes gum disease. The second is a hint on how to defeat gum disease: *Remove the plaque frequently so that the anaerobic bacteria do not have time to flourish under it and begin to cause problems.* We will talk about specific ways that plaque can be disrupted or removed soon.

As was just mentioned, dental plaque begins to reform virtually as soon as it is removed. It can sometimes be detected again within thirty minutes of removal. Therefore, the fight against gum disease is a never-ending dance. The plaque perpetually forms as you continue to remove it. Now, you can begin to realize why the problem of gum disease is so widespread. This is a constant ongoing battle that must be continuously fought. If more people understood this principle alone, perhaps there would be less suffering under the effects of gum disease. In addition, this is a war being fought against an invisible enemy. Since the enemy cannot be seen, it is that much more difficult to take the enemy seriously. Because most people do not realize they are fighting this type of ongoing war, they are not prepared to do what it takes to win.

Any gaps in the regular removal of plaque and the anaerobic bacteria hiding under it can lead to problems. Out of all the tooth and gum areas in your mouth, how can you be sure that you are getting it all? Even with daily removal of the plaque, you still need to be diligent about getting every potential spot that can harbor it. This adds another degree of complexity to solving the problem.

When plaque is not removed, the amount of bacteria under it continues to grow in number. When plaque ages, it hardens into tartar also known as calculus. As more toxins accumulate, the gum tissue begins to pull away from the tooth. The bacterial toxins along with the body's own enzymes, which are supposed to fight the bacteria, then begin to break down the connective tissues and the bone that supports the gums. You can probably surmise that things can continually worsen from this point on.

Moreover, most professionals generally agree that tartar cannot be removed at home, and needs a professional cleaning to be removed. If tartar is that strong, think how long the bacteria can grow there safely—perhaps as long as the time to your next professional cleaning. What about those who never go to the dentist? Uh-oh. You can imagine how serious this problem can get.

How many people understand these principles about gum disease? Among those who do have a basic understanding, how many consistently take daily action to fight or prevent it from occurring? The numbers arc miniscule in comparison to the general population. This is why I feel so strongly that greater public awareness is needed to help stop or mitigate the epidemic of gum disease. The dentist's office is one of the best places for awareness to be raised. Hopefully, this book will help, too.

We cannot put all the responsibility of fighting gum disease on dental professionals. People actually have to take action on their own when away from the dentist's office. Obviously, someone else cannot be there every day to disrupt the plaque for you. I believe more people will take action when they understand the problem correctly. The word needs to be spread. We all have a responsibility to be vigilant when it comes to our health care needs. It is a myth that your care providers can do it all for you.

Each of us needs to realize our own responsibilities.

Part of the trouble for the layperson is that it is fairly difficult to recognize one's own gum disease problems, especially in the early stages. For example, despite my own training in the life sciences, I was still unaware that a little bleeding from the gums during flossing, brushing, and dental cleanings was not normal. Rest assured there is nothing normal about bleeding gum tissue, not even when the bleeding is rather minute. In addition, your gums should not be sore when you floss them gently.

A case in point: A woman wrote in to my website regarding her symptoms. I noted carefully as she described what was going on, and I continually urged her to go the periodontist. As our conversation continued, she said that "it wasn't that bad" and only affected her front teeth. Based on what she had revealed, I had a feeling the situation was more severe. I continued to urge her to go to the periodontist until she finally did. She was astonished when she found out her problem was far worse and affected her whole mouth. I had endured a similar situation, so I was not caught off guard. Yet, it was an eye-opener for her. The moral of this story is you cannot assume you are free of problems until you are examined by a periodontist.

Many people rely exclusively on their dentist. I do not want you to miss this; both this woman and I had the same experience in that our dentists never referred us to the periodontist. We both referred ourselves. We both discovered that we had some serious stuff going on in our mouths. I do not know why the referrals were not forthcoming from our dentists. However, I do believe this problem of not referring patients to the periodontist is much more widespread than our two examples.

I recently spoke to a former hygienist who still works at a periodontist's office. She believed the reason for a lack of referrals was economically driven. Some dentists probably feel they can do the job themselves and retain the patient and the revenue stream that patient provides.

I can attest that my dentist did not clearly explain to me that bleeding gums during routine cleanings were not normal, and she also failed to tell me what to do about those bleeding gums. On top of that, she did not refer me out. If she had taken the time to explain in a complete way that I was having a problem and what it could lead to, I probably would have been motivated to learn more and take action earlier on. Just telling someone to brush and floss more and use a mouthwash does not explain the reasons why you should. It also does not explain the nature of the problem or what can happen if the problem is not corrected. Consequently, there is less motivation to follow such advice. I believe this lack of education about gum disease is a widespread problem that affects the majority of people.

Start to understand this problem and take greater action now. Saving your gums and teeth and thereby saving yourself expensive replacements is something that is largely in your hands. Going to the dentist once every six months without sufficient home care just is not good enough.

To be clear, my situation did not get as bad as some do. Luckily, I still have my teeth. However, I lost gum tissue. That is tissue that I would like to have kept. Therefore, I firmly believe that my dentist did not do the right thing by me. At the very least, she could have done more to inform me about what was going on in my mouth.

I know there are plenty of very good dentists who truly help and educate their patients. They also refer to other professionals, such as periodontists, when appropriate. I am not attempting to undermine the dental profession, but I am asserting that there are some practitioners who do not always do the best they can, both at educating and helping the patient.

Frankly, your gums and their interconnectedness to your body's health should be regarded and cared for with the greatest attention. There is no reason for a person not to be able to keep his or her natural teeth for a lifetime, barring accident or injury. There are very few exceptions to this. Yet, without the knowledge and motivation to do what is needed, gum health often deteriorates to the point of losing teeth.

Sometimes you have to take matters into your own hands. Do not wait for your dentist to tell you, because you could be waiting on a train that is never coming. Nike says, "Just Do It!" Well I say, "Go see a periodontist!" You will be better off in the end. There is no need to take any chances. Your periodontist can help you to fight gum disease and defeat it. Your dentist can too, but the periodontist is better prepared, more experienced, and better equipped for helping you with your gum health. Maybe since the periodontist is more focused on gum health, he or she ought to also be more in tune with what you need to improve the health of your gum tissue.

Your teeth and gums are far too precious to leave things to chance. If you are not already under the care of a dentist or peri-odontist, stop and make your appointment now. Do not start the next chapter until you have made your first appointment with a periodontist—if you are not currently under one's care.

*Do not consider painful
what is good for you.* —Euripedes

Professional Care

YOU PROBABLY REALIZE by now that failure to get professional help can spell disaster in so many ways. It is virtually impossible for most people to determine the state of their own gum health. It is normal for people to look themselves in the mirror every day, admiring their pearly whites, not realizing they are on the brink of disaster. This could go on for years. You might not even notice the problem until one day you realize your gums have receded and your teeth are loose. You see, gum disease is sneaky. It creeps in over time and gradually progresses so you get used to it before you even take notice of a difference. You could end up shouting the famous final plea: "How come I never noticed this before?"

In Chapter 1, I mentioned a woman whom I urged to visit the periodontist. She originally thought her gum disease problems were minor when, in fact, they were not at all. Situations like this illustrate why it is imperative that you visit a periodontist if you have or think you could have gum disease. The following conversation ensued after her visit.

My Response to an E-mail:

Ok, let me understand this correctly. You said that only your front 4 teeth are affected, right? Did he see more than that affected? In other words, is it more than your front teeth and is it really ALL of your gum tissue that is affected?

This is an important question. If your whole mouth is affected and you have tartar buildup under the gum line-well that could require a scaling and root planing.

That is the point when I started using the Hydro Floss. That worked for me and helped me avoid the SRP treatment. However, I cannot advise you to do what I did. Only your doctor should advise you or recommend treatment. Besides, he can see your mouth and I can't.

If only your front 4 teeth are affected, then I'm not sure about doing your whole mouth. If you are not sure or comfortable with your periodontist's recommendation, then you should get a second opinion. Otherwise, you are stuck following his treatment plan. However, it sounds to me like his opinion is that you have gum disease everywhere and not just on your front 4 teeth.

I do know what you meant by hyper sensitive-it hurts! It does sound like your problems are worse than you thought and mentioned to me.

Now, you have to decide whether you should get a second opinion or follow his treatment plan.

If you are going to have a scaling and root planing performed, you can't have it all done at once. It is not done that way. One side needs to heal up a bit before they do the other side.

It takes about 2 hours for each treatment.

I'm glad you went and got examined, it really sounds like it was worse than you thought / said it was.

Dave

Reader's Reply:

You are correct! I cannot see them, but I have pockets of red gums in between each and every tooth.

It is much worse than I thought, however I do not have bone loss YET! No loose teeth. I hate to even think of how painful this is going to be but I am tough—I will just have him do it!

I am not a dentist. I thought the few red gums were the bad part; well he used that long probe to check top pockets and several are more than 3mm.

He kept calling them out—it HURT!

So that tells me there is more going on in there! I said to heck with doing them all—you can see they are bad, just schedule me. Good thing my insurance covers 80%. So UNFORTUNATELY in one month unless any apts. are [scheduled] I go in for the worst cleaning ever! What happens to the gum when they pull them away from the tooth—would that mean they are more exposed? Do you have any literature about how it is done? GRRRRRRRRR. (BLUNTLY "THIS SUCKS")

SCARED TO DEATH

* * *

You can clearly see from this conversation that her thoughts about her problem and the true reality of the situation were a bit out of synch. Please, do not fool around with the health of your gums because you could lose one or more of your teeth. Even worse, you could also be harboring a chronic gum infection that is constantly feeding bacteria into your blood stream.

Though the evidence is not one hundred percent accepted yet, it is believed there is a correlation between gum disease and heart disease, stroke, and other illnesses in the body. Therefore, your gum health is indicative of the health of your body. Why do horse buyers look at a horse's teeth? This gives them an idea of the overall health of the horse. During the time of human slave trade, the teeth were also looked at the same way. This wisdom was ingrained in the society. They knew the health of the mouth reflected the health of the body.

You cannot allow fear of getting examined or having your teeth cleaned hold you back. If you are reading this book, it is possible that you already have gum disease. You *need* to have a professional evaluation done by a periodontist to tell you the current state of your gum health and what it will take to elevate that level of health, if necessary.

In addition, with that baseline evaluation, you will be able to tell if you are making real progress in the future when they reexamine you. They will use the measurements of pocket depth around each tooth to discover where your real problem areas are. Ask for those measurements. In the future, you will need that record to prove to yourself you have been making progress. If you have not made any progress, you will need to know that, as well.

These measurements will help you understand the extent of your problem.

- Anything beyond 3 mm is considered a problem.
- The number of 4 mm, 5 mm, and even greater pocket depth shows the relative health of your gums compared to what is considered normal.

This chapter comes before the chapter on home care because if you have—or think you might have—gum disease; professional care is the first step. You are forbidden from reading the next chapter on home care until you receive an evaluation, diagnosis, and treatment plan from a periodontist.

If you are not under the care of a periodontist right at this moment, then stop what you are doing and make an appointment right now. If it is after business hours and no offices are open, bookmark this page and do not read further until you have made that appointment.

Go ahead, I will wait right here.
...waiting...
...waiting...

Done? If your answer is yes: Good! Read on!

If you have not made that appointment yet, do not read any further until you do. The health of your gums is no joke and should not be taken lightly. You absolutely do not want to lose any teeth if it can be avoided. The Mayo Clinic founder suggested that *losing your teeth would shorten your life by ten years.*

If you still are not convinced that you need professional care for you gums and teeth, then I do not know what else to say.

Find a Professional You Can Trust
The quality of care you receive from professionals is very important. It is important that you like and trust your periodontist, dentist, or any other health care professional. Let me tell you a story to illustrate this point:

Picture yourself sitting in the dentist's chair and your dentist says to you, "That looks a little sticky. I think we need to drill into that and see how far the problem goes. We could start right away." Being conservative about such things, you might find yourself responding, "What exactly is wrong?" The answer is less than confidence inspiring: "Well, it might be a cavity."

"Might?" you inquire. "It could be reversible or irreversible pulpitis. We like to practice preventive dentistry here so I think we should drill it and fill it, just to be safe."

Fortunately, even though she was talking pretty fast at this point, you managed to hear the phrase "reversible pulpitis." You make a mental note of that. Despite the dentist's repeated requests to schedule an appointment to get that tooth filled, you manage to escape without making any promises or creating any friction. As you drive home, the word "reversible" repeats itself in your mind. After arriving home, you do an Internet search for the term "reversible pulpitis," and what you discover shocks you. The prognosis for reversible pulpitis is good *without* intervention.

Upon further investigation, you learn that the dental enamel in your teeth is constantly in a state of flux. It gets soft and then hard again. This dance of enamel hardening and softening is ongoing. Reversible pulpitis may or may not develop into a cavity.

Sound like a strange story to you? It is a true story that happened to me. Naturally, I was not happy with the level of service provided by that dentist, and I stopped visiting her. Safeguarding our health is the duty of every health care practitioner. I avoid practitioners who are not reasonably honoring that code to the best of their ability.

I learned that eating hard cheese and/or using a fluoride rinse can help the enamel to harden again. Many popular soft drinks and sugary substances can really weaken tooth enamel and make it soft and ripe for a cavity. When the problem enters the realm of *irreversible*, you truly have a cavity that needs to be filled—but not before then.

I never went back to that dentist. When I visited a new dentist six months later, there was no sign of any cavity. Had I listened to the first dentist, she would have put another hole in a perfectly good tooth and filled it with a substance that was not natural to my mouth. It would have stayed there for the rest of my life. That is, if it did not need to be replaced twenty years from now.

I would like to take a moment to remind you that I am not a dental professional. I am just an average person who has spent a lot of time researching these issues and terms in order to become as knowledgeable as I can about how to safeguard my health.

That said, I want to share with you a post that was sent in to my blog recently from a dental professional named Sue. While I hope this will show how a lot of medical information you can get out there is up for debate, keep in mind that any information I share in this book is true to the best of my knowledge based on my own experiences and research.

Sue wrote:

I am a dentist, and your description of reversible pulpitis is incorrect.

What you are actually describing is arrested caries. Reversible pulpitis is inflammation of the pulpal tissue [soft tissue inside the tooth including nerves and blood vessels] that is caused by an irritant. Once the irritant is removed, the pulpitis (inflammation) will resolve.

Arrested decay occurs when tooth structure begins the decay process, and because of certain factors (lack of substrate, fluoridation treatments) the caries can be halted, or arrested.

This area can be remineralized with the calcium from within the saliva, or fluoride. The evidence of arrested decay is seen radiographically as an area that is not progressing.

However, that requires multiple radiographs taken 6 months apart to visualize the progress.

My Reply:
Thank you, Sue.

I do truly appreciate your correction. I will tell you why I refer to reversible pulpitis the way I do. When my dentist tried to drill a perfectly good tooth and I questioned her about it, she said, "It could be reversible pulpitis."

I'm sure that your correction is accurate, but I am also equally sure that the situation I described previously is widely referred to as reversible pulpitis by dental professionals. I am certain of this because I described the situation I experienced as "reversible pulpitis" on multiple occasions to dental professionals, including dentists and hygienists, and not one of them corrected me on my usage of the term.

Perhaps this is one of those terms that has fallen into misuse as do so many other words from professional or lay literature?

Here is information on pulpitis as taken from Wikipedia [Wikipedia.org]:

Causes of Pulpitis

1. Caries that penetrate though the tooth enamel, the dentin, and into the pulp.

2. Repeated dental procedures or tooth trauma

Thanks again, Sue. If you could share more insight on this, it would be greatly appreciated.

Dave

✻ ✻ ✻

When I was only about nineteen years old, I was stationed on a naval base in Maryland. I went to visit a dentist there. He examined my mouth and said that I needed a gum graft. Keep in mind how young I was. I was also less cynical and more trusting than I am now. It is not good to be overly cynical, but sometimes a healthy dose provides a little extra protection in this crazy world.

At any rate, this dentist told me I needed a gum graft. I agreed, although I was a little anxious about the whole scenario. He completed the graft, and I went back two weeks later for an evaluation. He announced that the graft did not take and asked me if I wanted to try again. That made me a little nervous. Why would he ask me that? Didn't he know if it needed to be done again or not? My alarm bells sounded. I said no. I was a little perturbed as I began to realize what had happened. His assistant came into the room. I think she could read my reactions quite well, and she confided in me. She told me that this dentist had just learned this procedure at a nearby naval hospital.

I was appalled.

Fast-forward a few years to when I was twenty-three years old. I was fresh out of the navy and taking classes at a local community college. I was living at home at the time and went to visit the dentist I used to go to before joining the navy. My mother held this particular dentist in high regard. When he came in to examine my mouth, he asked me if I was having any problems. I told him there was a certain area of my mouth where I was feeling a bit of pain.

He looked in my mouth for about five to ten seconds. Then he said two sentences that just do not belong together: "I don't see anything wrong. We could do a root canal." In defense of the dentist, maybe he was joking with me. I do not know. But I do know that kind of joke should not be made during an examination.

At this point, the warning flags went up. I was a little wiser after my previous experience. I recognized immediately the absurdity of those two phrases being used in conjunction. I said no. Two weeks later, the pain I was experiencing disappeared and never came back again. It has been about fifteen years since then. If there had been a real problem, I would have known by now. I have also had a number of x-rays since then and many dentists have examined me. No one has ever noticed any problem that might warrant a root canal. I have never needed a root canal to date.

A root canal would kill the tooth—if the tooth was not already dead—by carving out the nerve that supplies it. The tooth will die and turn brown. This marks the need for a crown, which is an additional expense. I am so glad that I did not blindly submit to a root canal I did not need.

I am not alone in these experiences. I ran into a woman who told me that one dentist told her she had five or six cavities. She went to another dentist who said she had none. Who was telling the truth? The second dentist would not likely say there were no cavities if there really were some there. However, the first dentist could have been motivated by revenue. You possibly have your own stories, or have heard the stories of friends and relatives who will tell you to be careful when choosing a professional.

You could be wondering why I took the time to relate these true stories. I want to illustrate the point that professional care is only as effective as the practitioner. If a practitioner is willing to make money from "gray," or questionable areas, then he/she is not looking out for the patient's best interests. After all, human beings are "only human," and as much as we want to put our medical and dental professionals on the pedestal of unquestionable integrity, common sense tells us that would be a bad idea.

The only way to reduce your chances of being a victim of unethical action is to be an educated, informed patient. No one is going to give you that education, so it is important that you go after the information yourself. By reading this book, you are taking a step in the right direction.

In the case of the first story, how many people would have let the dentist start right away? I am willing to go out on a limb and say that the majority of dental patients would have. As you know, this lack of questioning could lead to some dangerous and costly situations.

Let me reiterate that I am not here to bash any profession. I respect the various specialties and fields within the health care industry. I am just reminding you that there are bad apples in every bunch and you need to look out for them. I have an excellent periodontist, and I am very pleased with his services. What I am advocating is that you develop the sensitivity to find a good dentist or periodontist and develop the wisdom to know the difference when you run into one who adheres to less than the highest ethical standards.

Here are some suggestions: Ask a lot of questions. Pay close attention to what your health care practitioner says and how he or she responds. If your dentist does not have time to answer all your questions thoroughly and patiently, then you might consider moving on. I would much rather be cared for by someone who is genuinely concerned about my health more than the bottom line numbers of the business. Besides, you are paying for these services. Your dentist's reaction to your questions is a telltale sign. Pay close attention.

You will have to weigh your practitioner's time crunch against your need for information and getting your questions answered, and then decide if you are getting the level of care you deserve. There are doctors, dentists, and periodontists who will take the time to patiently answer all your questions, though it might be a little difficult to find one. Your health is arguably your most precious asset. Do what you must to safeguard it. If that means "firing" your dentist and finding another one, then maybe that is what you should do.

High-caliber dental care providers should actually appreciate your questions. They should be pleased when you show a willingness to take part in your own dental care. Compare the informative, appreciative providers to those who seem aloof and do not take the time to help you understand every nuance of your health and its maintenance. Which would you prefer to work with? Dentists can only do so much from the office, and all of them understand the need for you to take appropriate measures at home. A dental professional who is willing to give you all the information you need to make his or her job easier is a wise person.

When you are asking questions, take notes, written or mental, and then research the information again later for a clearer idea about what is going on. Each time you do so, you will probably have more questions for your caregiver at your next visit.

If you are working with someone who is tolerant of your questions and patiently answers them, providing you with new information each time, you will come away with an empowered feeling. You will be much more knowledgeable and less anxious about your situation. Seek out those providers who are willing to empower you in this way.

Second Opinions

Have you ever questioned a diagnosis or treatment plan that your health care provider has suggested? If you have misgivings about your care provider's diagnosis or treatment, you have the right to seek a second opinion. Imagine how you would feel if you ignored your gut instinct to get a second opinion only to find out later that your health care provider was not acting in your best interest. Your health is precious, so do not fool around, and try not to cut corners.

Basically, you should not leave a practitioner's office with big questions on your mind, any more than you should leave with doubts or suspicions. If you do, those doubts all need to be answered for a couple of reasons. You need to feel comfortable with what is going on. You need this for both your own sanity and to help insure that you follow the treatment plan and home care recommendations your care provider makes. If you have unanswered questions, it is easy to lose the motivation to maintain a home care regimen.

I have had several other less than ideal encounters with caregivers. I do not revisit the ones I have bad experiences with. As a corollary to this, if you seek out people who have a high degree of morals and ethics in any aspect of life, you are probably going to have more enjoyable and higher quality experiences. Yet, all human beings are fallible, and one should never lose sight of this fact.

Despite the above stories, you should really view your periodontist or dentist as your friend in the fight against gum disease. They can do things to help you that you can not do on your own.

If you already know that you have gum disease, as I mentioned before, you should seek the services of a periodontist. If you have lost too much of your gum tissue and/or supporting bone structure underneath, they might be able to partially rebuild it through surgery. Once your gum tissue has been restored, you will learn how to keep it healthy for the rest of your life through a combination of great home care and professional care. Since this surgical process could be time consuming, costly, and painful, you will naturally want to do everything you can to insure that your gum tissue remains healthy in the future.

It is also possible that the periodontist will determine you do not need any such procedures at all. Won't it feel good to know the exact state of your gum health so you do not have to constantly speculate or worry about your situation?

Of course, gum disease is not the only thing that erodes your gum tissue. You also need to be wary of brushing too hard because your gums can be damaged as a result. The biofilm called dental plaque is fragile. When you brush, it is only the plaque you are attempting to eradicate. Therefore, there is no reason to brush hard. You will do a better job brushing gently. Remember that your goal is to clean away the plaque while preserving your gum tissue. Tartar, a.k.a calculus, could be another story. Tartar could require professional cleaning to remove. How can you tell the difference? That is what your dentist or periodontist is for.

The Need for Regular Dental Cleanings
Aside from keeping a wary eye on the state of your gum health or disease, one of the biggest benefits to seeing your periodontist is the dental cleanings. These do more than just keep the stains off your teeth. They also help protect the health of your gums. I have

had my teeth cleaned in dentists' offices all my life, but when I had my first cleaning in a periodontist's office, it proved to be head and shoulders above the regular cleaning in a dentist's office. Unfortunately, I cannot give you a super logical explanation or argument for this—it was just better. As one hygienist in the periodontist's office told me, the focus is just a little different during the cleanings.

Most people think it is sufficient to have their teeth professionally cleaned about once every six months. Somehow, six-month cleanings have become the standard by which insurance pays (or does not pay) for care. Your dentist or periodontist can sometimes write a persuasive letter asking insurance companies to pay for cleanings every three months. There is evidence that supports the notion that three-month cleanings are more effective than six-months for the prevention of gum disease.

If you have not been to a dentist for a very long time, they will probably want you to start off with a solid cleaning after your initial examination. If it has been a while, there is likely to be a lot of built-up plaque and tartar. This buildup needs to be removed, because it is precisely the plaque and tartar that harbors the anaerobic bacteria that cause gum disease. It is something that brushing alone cannot combat. Once you are getting your teeth cleaned professionally on a regular basis, it will be much easier for your home care to be meaningful and effective.

I suppose that if you were a trained professional, you would be able to scale your own teeth. Even in that case, it is still better to let someone else do it in order to get the spots you might overlook.

There have been a number of studies done on the effects of frequency of professional cleanings. The concept of six-month cleanings that you are probably familiar with was created from a very old study that only considered the health of the teeth, not the gums. Due to a number of factors that influence the standard of care, the six-month cleaning interval persists in the dental industry. It is, however, in many cases, not good enough to support the health of your gums to an optimal degree.

I prefer a professional dental cleaning every two months. This might seem a little excessive, but trust me, it is not. Many people see dental cleanings as nothing more than a little scraping and an opportunity to see shiny and sophisticated instruments at work. However, professional cleanings have great value in your fight to prevent gum disease.

If your periodontist agrees that you should have two-month cleanings, you will likely have to pay for it out-of-pocket. The chances of your insurance company picking up the bill are slim to none. However, I reason that it is worth the additional expense for the extra protection to my gum health.

Scaling and Root Planing (SRP)

These treatments are also referred to as root scaling and planing. You can hear these terms used interchangeably, but they mean the same thing. Never allow terminology or jargon in the dentist or periodontist's office to get in your way of understanding what is going on.

SRP is drastically different from your regular dental cleanings. Scaling and root planings are much deeper cleanings that normally involve a local anaesthetic and additional work. The hygienist will scrape down along the root to remove rough spots that provide fertile ground for tartar build up as well as remove the tartar itself. The treatment is usually done in multiple visits because it takes about two hours to treat half of your mouth. The goal of doing a scaling and root planing is to have it done only once. With proper home care and professional maintenance, the need for second and third treatments should be minimal. Unfortunately, there are people who need SRP treatments more than once.

Remember the story I told you before? You know, when I decided to go out on my own after I was told I needed an SRP treatment? Instead of getting one, I went out and purchased a Hydro Floss. After using it for about five months, I was told I no longer needed a root scaling and planing. While I do not make any guarantee about the effectiveness of the Hydro Floss, I can say that it worked for me. You might not experience the same results that I did, so it is best to follow the treatment plan of your care provider. Do not take risks with your dental health.

You can read more about the Hydro Floss at:
http://www.ToBeInformed.com/hydrofloss

Should you decide to purchase a Hydro Floss there, you can use coupon code **A-PER10** at checkout to score free ground shipping in the United States and a free tube of PerioTherapy toothpaste. We will talk about that toothpaste more in Chapter 3.

The Hydro Floss at the above address also comes with AktivOxigen Serum. You can read more about what AktivOxigen is and does at: http://tobeinformed.com/oxygen-serum

Since I found a way to avoid root scaling and planing treatment, I do not have any first-hand stories to tell you about what one is like. However, one of the readers of my site had the procedure done.

Here is what she had to say:

UPDATE!

Half of my mouth was scaled and to be honest it was NOT as bad as I thought!

No bone loss or buildup. He thinks I might have an allergy to my own gums. We did decide to go ahead with the 3 month cleanings and so fourth. I go back next Tues. to get it done on the other side of my mouth.

It is not bad at all!

I am on Chlorhexidine every other month but for 2 weeks. So that pretty much sums it up! I am all for the scaling—it is not as bad as it sounds!

More later when I get some time.

My Reply:
Hi Heather,

This is great news! I'm very glad that you are now under professional care and have been given a game plan to stop the progression of gum disease and keep it under control from here on out.

It is very good news to hear that you don't have any bone loss.

I'm glad that your experience was a positive one. As I mentioned before, my sister seemed very unhappy with the treatment.

It's good for the other readers of this site to understand that it can be a very positive experience.
Please continue to keep us updated!

Dave

Her next update:
Dave and all;

Second half was not so bad. She could not see any buildup under the gum line.

I did learn a valuable thing, this might seem silly, USE HOT WATER to make your tooth brush soft, add the paste then brush, this ensures the tooth brush stays soft and you do not damage your gums. Neat trick, huh?

Anyhow, the second scaling was easy! Not even a shot! Yeah you heard me... it was not bad at all. I feel it is not a bad procedure and would really encourage anyone needing it done to go for it!! It is not as scary and bad as it seems! I had a gum scaling and root scaling as well. Nothing!

So that being said, if you need it GO get it done—then it is recommended you get your teeth cleaned every 3 months. It cost me $100.00 out of pocket for the ones not insured (the 6 month cleanings) so really not bad and so worth it!

If it will save my gums I am going for it! So Best of luck to you all and I also encourage you to use Dr Katz products and the Hydro Floss—they are very good in prevention!

Good luck to you all!

More to come!

Back in a month for a checkup!

Heather

My Reply:
Thank you Heather. This is exactly the kind of thing people need to hear about. Please keep us posted.

You can get a free downloadable copy of Dr. Katz's book, The Bad Breath Bible, *at:* Tobeinformed.com/bbbook. *This is a $10 value according to his site.*

❊   ❊   ❊

Giving Your Gum Health a Boost

Here is a little trick to give your gum health a little boost. You will have to get your dentist or periodontist to cooperate for this to work. Chlorhexidine is a prescription mouthwash that is excellent for clearing up the bacteria that are responsible for harming your gum tissue.

However, it has the side effect of staining your teeth. It can also destroy the normal bacterial balance in your mouth. If your dentist or periodontist agrees and actually writes the prescription for you, you could use it for a week or two weeks before your next professional cleaning. The cleaning will remove any stain that the use of chlorhexidine might produce. Obviously, this should only be done under the guidance of your dentist or doctor.

Chlorhexidine is not appropriate and is probably not going to be prescribed for long term use. Here is an interesting note that a hygienist sent in:

Hi Dave,

Just checked in and read a little on your website and the comment about Chlorhexidine caught my eye. In my opinion, Chlorhexidine is NOT for long term use.... Generally I have been taught to recommend it for only 7-10 days post treatment for Scaling and Root Planing (SRP) then to switch to Listerine or Crest Oral Health for over the counter daily care.

Chlorhexidine is too powerful for long term use and wipes out all the flora in the mouth to throw off the natural balance. The stain, of course, is a problem, but more than that, Chlorhexidine can also cause an increase in dental tartar accumulation which in turn will make it increasingly difficult for the patient to keep out the plaque...downward spiral...etc, etc...

Also, I know you recommend patients see a periodontist if they think they have periodontal disease. I do think you can also get good care in a general practice, if there is a hygienist who is taking time and care to do a periodontal exam and is skilled in expanded periodontal treatment.

It can be more cost effective for people to get their conservative periodontal treatment in a general dentist's office rather than a specialist (Periodontist) practice.

I hope I am not stepping on any toes, but these are some of my thoughts. All best.. you are doing a great job getting the word out! Congratulations to Heather and all that she is doing to improve her health!

Sincerely,
Hillary, RDH, BSDH

*Note: I believe she meant to say Crest *Pro*-Health

* * *

Since chlorhexidine isn't going to be a good long-term solution, you might want to take a look at the "mouthwash cocktail" section in Chapter 3 of this book. This is a series of three common mouthwashes you can purchase at virtually any drug store without a prescription.

Periodontal Surgery
There are different kinds of periodontal surgery. As mentioned before, if you have suffered moderate to severe gum disease, you

could need some restorative work done. Your periodontist will probably let you know what, if any, work he or she recommends after your initial evaluation.

I was happy to discover that my gums were not in terribly bad shape, but there was one area that needed some tissue added. I was told that it was not critical, but that it was a good idea. I probably could have gotten away without the gum graft, but I felt that it would not hurt and would make me feel like I had a safety net for the tissue that supports that tooth.

I am going to share my experience in order to give you an idea of what you might expect should you need to have any periodontal surgery done. I also want to deflate any fears you might have about getting such a procedure done. I understand that for many people, just visiting the dentist for a routine exam and cleaning is terrifying, let alone actually having any surgery done.

Hopefully, you have been instilled with enough knowledge and experiences that you realize not having professional care puts you in a more fearful situation. If not, that is something you will definitely have to overcome. Let's put it into perspective: If I can sit through this surgery and go to work the same day, it is not that bad.

Here is the story of my dental surgery.

I arrive at the office four minutes before 8:00 am. They tell me they are ready for me and sit me in a chair. Then, the assistant informs me that the doctor has just arrived in the parking lot. Since I have worked with him before, I know that he is really confident and competent, so I do not sweat this too much. I am thankful for our trusting relationship, because if I had not been feeling comfortable, the announcement that the doctor was late could have added to any anxiety I might have been feeling.

The doctor arrives and says a few pleasant words and then gets down to business. There are two areas that need to be numbed; one is on the roof of my mouth. This is where the donor tissue comes from. The other was on the labial area of tooth # 28. (Labial = lip side as opposed to the lingual or tongue side of the tooth.) They numb the aforementioned areas of my mouth with a drug called Articaine. I have always been highly tolerant of needles in the mouth, so the little pricks do not bother me much.

I am really surprised at how quickly the Articaine takes effect. They only wait about five minutes before starting the procedure. Since the doctor wears glasses I can see what he is doing through the reflection. I decide to close my eyes. I am not that keen on seeing my own blood. I do not know anyone who is. Besides, I want to take my mind off the actual work he is doing, and I do not want to flinch.

They use gauze and a suction device, and they are so proficient and skillful that I do not detect a single drop of blood hitting the back of my throat.

The idea of the surgery was to replace tissue lost to gum disease and/or brushing too hard. The doctor applies some stitches on the tooth # 28 area that will not dissolve. He also uses dissolvable stitches on the roof of my mouth along with dissolvable gauze that will disappear in about four days.

Since it is not possible to perform normal home care in the area involving the surgery for a few days, I am given a prescription for a chlorhexidine rinse to kill the bacteria that can produce gum disease or infection. He also gives me a prescription for a systemic (taken internally) antibiotic—Doxycycline (100) mg—to be taken every twelve hours, also to prevent infection.

The doctor gives me some ice packs to apply right after the surgery. I continue to ice five to fifteen minutes on and five minutes off until about 3:00 in the afternoon. (The procedure was performed around 8:00 am.)

The most astonishing thing about the ordeal is that after visiting the local pharmacy to get my prescriptions filled, I actually proceed to work after the surgery. I get home from work exhausted, and I sleep from the time I arrive home until the next morning.

I even decide to forgo the painkillers because the pain is not severe enough to bother with the pills.

A week later, the doctor removes the stitches. He says that I should expect minor bleeding for the next four days when I clean the area with a swab of chlorhexidine. He says the bleeding will stop, and I should begin gently brushing the area. Surprisingly, I never experience any bleeding after the removal of the stitches.

Overall, I was pleased with the amount of tissue that was restored. I walked away with some cushion against further gum recession. That area of my mouth seemed healthier and even more youthful.

Considering I went to work the same morning and did not use the painkillers, we can conclude that this was a very minor surgery. I was one of the lucky ones this time, and I do not take that for granted

Although I experienced a relatively smooth process, I urge you to protect and nurture your gum tissue so you will never need a surgery like this one. If it is too late for that and you do need surgery, remember that if I could go to work right after the procedure, it was not too bad.

Of course, more advanced problems could possibly require insertion of bone matrix or some other similar techniques. These procedures might require more recovery time. My boss had something like that done and it did not seem to keep her from work for very long, either. Your periodontist can tell you what you need and what to expect in terms of recovery.

There you have it, my experience with gum surgery! It was not the end of the world after all.

Remember, even gum grafts might not do everything you would like them to; the results could be far less than you expect. Keep this in mind when considering your options for surgery.

Here is something I reported on my blog about two and a half weeks after the surgery. This can help give you an idea of what to expect:

> *It has now been about two and one-half weeks since my gum graft surgery was performed.*
>
> *The results have been pretty good. I was hoping for the gum tissue to settle a little higher but it is still pretty good.*
>
> *The reason I had gum surgery was gum recession. It seems likely that the recession was due more to brushing too hard than to gum disease. Though, diseased gum tissue is certainly weaker than healthy tissue.*
>
> *In either case, the periodontist said this was the only spot that needed some work. My gums are healthy and pink and they are not diseased at this point, but years of brushing too hard have left my gums receded.*

The purpose of brushing is little more than to remove a thin biofilm called plaque that houses the anaerobic bacteria that cause gum disease and cavities.

The biofilm is very weak. Yet, to prevent gum disease, it must be removed daily. That is the purpose of brushing and flossing.

*Since the biofilm is weak, **there is NO REASON to ever brush hard**. Instead brush very gently. See your periodontist or hygienist for specific directions on brushing and flossing.*

You need both home care and professional care. You cannot get by on either alone, you need both. For the professional care of your gums, it is best to see a periodontist. (Oh, did I say that already??)

✴ ✴ ✴

Bruxism (Grinding Your Teeth) and Custom Dental Guards
I have added this bit of information about grinding your teeth and custom dental guards under the professional care section because custom-made dental guards are fitted by a dentist. If you grind your teeth, getting one of these could be worth your while.

Some people believe they can get by with the moldable variety that you get in the drug store or even in sporting goods stores. You make this type at home by dipping the guard in very hot water and molding it to your teeth.

If you look carefully on the packaging, you will see that they usually say not to use them for more than a few months. If you are grinding your teeth, you probably should get a professionally made and molded dental guard.

I found the difference between the drug store and custom made variety to be pretty vast. One of the nice things about the custom-made guard is that it snaps snuggly into place around your upper teeth and you will not spit it out at night. Unfortunately, the home molded kind tends to end up outside your mouth before morning comes—which, of course, negates the purpose of using a mouth guard in the first place.

The downside of the custom, professionally made guards is that they are expensive. When I had mine made just a short while before writing this, it cost me over five hundred dollars. However, I think it was worth it. I view it as spending the money on the front end to save pain and money in the future.

In addition to the cost, I have also had to go in for additional adjustments and I am looking at going in again. It is very important for the custom guard to fit properly. If it does not, you can wake up with aching teeth as a result of extreme pressure concentrated on a few teeth. This pain defeats the purpose of preventing grinding with a mouth guard.

Grinding the teeth is something that should be stopped. You do not want to wear your teeth down to tiny studs, do you? In addition, the high pressure created from teeth grinding can cause damage to the supporting structure beneath the gums. If you have gum disease, this can add to the destruction of the already weakened and taxed tissue. If you grind your teeth while sleeping, be sure to check with your doctor about getting a custom mouth guard.

I can still feel a couple of spots in my mouth where the teeth have become smooth instead of having natural ridges that are essential for grinding and rending food. Had I gotten a guard made earlier, this erosion would probably have been prevented. The tooth erosion does not currently cause me any noticeable problems, but I prefer to protect what I have.

As I mentioned before, I have had to get my custom guard adjusted several times. If you get one, this is a normal part of the process. It is important to get the guard to fit properly to prevent more problems. Generally, the dentist will use a tool to custom shape your guard. He will try to get it to a point where the pressure is evenly distributed so that no part of your mouth or teeth encounters undue stress from wearing it.

If there is a tooth or section of teeth that is pressing on the guard more than others, you will feel the pressure in that area when you wake up in the morning. If this happens, call the dentist and get him/her to adjust your guard. Once you pay the initial fee for having the mold made, you should not have to pay for adjustments.

The problem of getting the mouth guard adjusted is complicated by the fact that your jaw may actually start to relax more to the fit of the guard over time. This is normal. However, it can bring the necessity for additional adjustments because the points that are touching the guard have shifted.

The goal of adjusting the guard is to get all your teeth to touch evenly. When that happens, you will feel really good about wearing the guard. It will not be noticeable when you sleep and it will not inadvertently slip out of your mouth during the night. Overall, it was well worth it to get the custom guard made.

Force has no place
where there is need of skill —Herodotus

Home Care

Good Home Care is Essential

HOME CARE IS very important in maintaining the health of your gum tissue. However, I cannot repeat enough that it is to be utilized in conjunction with professional care, not in place of it. You need both professional care and home care; the value of one is greatly diminished without the other.

As mentioned previously, dental plaque is the culprit responsible for creating gum disease. More accurately, it creates a habitat for the anaerobic bacteria that secrete the toxins that harm your gum tissue and dental enamel. Those little beasts never rest. They keep on reproducing. Remember, this is a battle that must be fought every day.

There is a rare two percent of the population which seems to have a natural immunity to gum disease. They are the lucky ones. Chances are pretty high that you are in the other ninety-eight percent, as am I. Therefore, you really need to do a good job at home care.

Plaque is a multi-headed, regenerating monster. It attacks your entire mouth simultaneously and it begins to reform immediately after being disrupted. It can be detectable again within thirty minutes of removal, so you will have to be diligent. It is the same whether you are already suffering from gum disease or just want to prevent it in the first place.

Disrupting the plaque frequently is what we are talking about when discussing home care. Now that you know what home care is for, let's talk about what kind of tools, products, and techniques you might use at home to help you defeat plaque and the anaerobic bacteria that cause gum disease and tooth decay.

A Word about pH and Your Mouth

Do not underestimate the importance of pH in the mouth. Bacteria love an acidic environment; it gets them excited and causes those colonies to grow even more quickly, secrete more acids, and cause more damage. Therefore, we want to deprive them of an acidic environment to the greatest extent possible.

PH refers to the phrase "power of hydrogen." To illustrate, imagine—just for a moment—bathing your teeth in acid. As you can surmise, acid is bad for your teeth. This is because acid can pull minerals right out of them, making your teeth weaker and more prone to cavities. Bacteria, the kind that cause cavities and gum disease, secrete acids that damage our enamel and irritate our gums.

These nasty little critters like your mouth to be more acidic. They love that type of environment and it helps to nurture them. They do not like the opposite, which would be called an alkaline, or basic environment.

In addition, there are some foods and drinks that we put in our mouths that directly attack our teeth. Abstaining from these substances would be a great idea, but perhaps not very practical. So, we need to alter the pH of our mouths as soon as possible after or even while we are consuming such things. If you are prone to cavities, then this is going to be even more important to you.

Imagine a scale from 0 to 14. Anything below 7 on that scale is considered acidic, and anything above 7 would be alkaline. The mouth hovers around 7 and doesn't generally go below 6.3. If it does, this can definitely contribute to the problems we just talked about. But, some people have so much dental plaque secreting acids that it can actually make the mouth pH even lower than 6.3 on a regular basis! Now that is scary! Imagine constantly staying in that state. The enamel on your teeth would not last very long. As you might guess, this state could cause you to get more cavities and contribute to the progression of gum disease. Yikes!

Your saliva acts as a *buffer*. A buffer, in this case, is nothing more than something that causes the pH to move towards seven—the neutral factor on the pH scale.

Have you ever heard of someone using lemon juice to whiten his or her teeth? *This is a very bad idea.* Do not do it. Basically, you would be brushing your teeth with acid!

The reason I bring this up is to help you pay attention to what kind of mouthwash you use. If you use a mouthwash that is on the acidic side, then you do not want to brush your teeth right after because you would be brushing the acid into your teeth, accelerating the weakening process.

How can you tell if a mouthwash is acidic or alkaline (basic)? Usually, mouthwashes that are not acidic like to brag about it. You will see something on the label that says "mild pH." They are trying to tell you that they are alkaline, the opposite of acidic—or at least close to neutral. That is a good thing when it comes to oral hygiene. The mouthwashes that are acidic are not likely to advertise that fact.

Therefore, if you do not see anything on the label indicating pH, you will need to call the company and ask them. That is the best way. Now, if you want to get fancy, you could get some pH strips and stick them in the liquid you are trying to test. The strip will turn a certain color and you will look on the scale that comes with the strip to see what pH that color equates to. However, that seems like a lot of trouble. It is easier to pick a mouthwash that says "mild pH," or just use your phone; call the company that makes the mouthwash and *ask*.

If you do use something acidic on your mouth, then immediately follow up with something alkaline to protect your tooth enamel and help to create an environment that is friendly to you, but not to the nasty little critters we call bacteria. Chewing xylitol gum can do the trick. You will be reading about xylitol soon. At the very least, you can rinse your mouth with water after putting something acidic in your mouth. Water generally has a neutral pH. (Seven is the number that denotes neutral on the pH scale.) You could sip water with foods or drinks that are acidic in nature. After drinking something acidic, if you have no other method available to raise pH, at the very least, vigorously rinse your mouth with water.

For example, if you drink a very acidic, phosphoric acid-containing drink such as many popular soft drinks, you are essentially bathing your teeth in acid. If at all possible, rinse your mouth out with water after drinking such powerfully acidic substances. It would be a good idea to chew some xylitol gum after that and/or rinse with a mouthwash that has a mild pH. There are many foods and drinks that are acidic. You would probably be able to find a chart or two on the Internet.

The important point to all this is that after using or eating something acidic in our mouths, we want to drive the pH a bit higher to compensate. The purpose is both to inhibit bacteria and to protect our tooth enamel from corrosion. If you are familiar with balancing the pH in a fish tank, just consider your mouth to be a similar environment. Saltwater fish will die if the water becomes too acidic. In the same sense, we want to keep our mouths as close to neutral as we can, generally speaking. With a higher pH, your body's natural way of making the teeth stronger can function, thereby helping to protect you from cavities as well as slowing down the proliferation of those little monsters we call bacteria.

So what are some mouthwashes that have a mild pH, meaning that they are slightly alkaline or at least close to neutral, instead of acidic? You could take a jaunt to your local drug store and search the labels. I know that CLÖSYS is a good one and should be right there on the shelf. It also happens to be part of a very powerful mouthwash combination I have dubbed "The Mouthwash Cocktail." You will be reading more about it very soon.

I also know that all of the mouthwashes Dr. Katz has created are of a slightly alkaline pH. If you have access to the Internet, you can see all of them here:

http://tobeinformed.com/mw

One of the reasons I brought this up so early in the chapter on home care is because you are going to be presented with a bunch of cool tools, products, and techniques that could help improve your dental health. The question is going to come up at some point, "When do I brush, before or after doing [fill in the blank]?" Following the line of reasoning presented in this section, you would want to brush or use other tools when your mouth is closer to a neutral or even slightly alkaline pH.

For example, virtually everyone is familiar with a popular mouthwash that contains a lot of alcohol. Brushing directly after using it, without doing something to move your mouth closer to a neutral pH might not be the best for your dental health. Remember the example of brushing with lemon juice? While this mouthwash might not be quite that bad, you probably get the idea.

On the other hand, just last night I talked to a man who told me he has used such a mouthwash for ten years without worrying about pH and has never had a problem. We want to do what is optimal for our dental health and we might not have the same unique experience this man had.

I did a little experiment measuring pH and I would like to share my results with you. The values given are approximated from a color chart that came with the strips. I did not have a precision instrument to gauge the exact pH, and I did not take multiple readings for an average. Therefore, if you were to repeat my tests, you would likely come up with slightly different results. Here are the results that I obtained from testing some liquids with pH strips:

CLÖSYS: 7.2-7.4

Listerine: 5.8-6.0

My saliva after waking up: 6.4 [not ideal]

My saliva after chewing xylitol gum: 8.0 [You will be reading more about xylitol shortly.]

Brushing and Flossing – Still Essential

First, we will discuss brushing and flossing; those are the mechanical plaque-disrupting methods most people are familiar with. While very important, remember that they alone might not be enough to stop the development or progress of gum disease. Some could debate whether the problem is with brushing and flossing or the way they are being done. Still, there is just too much dental disease—both gum disease and cavities—for us to say that brushing and flossing alone do the job properly.

I find it interesting that the pat answer to patients in dental offices is that they need to brush or floss more to stop their growing problems. I wonder how often such advice is of practical benefit to the patients? How often, or in how many cases, does such advice stop or prevent gum disease? I doubt there has been a study on that exact question, but I think I already know the answer. I am willing to bet there are a ton of people who brush and floss like crazy and still get both cavities and/or gum disease.

Both brushing and flossing are important and you should definitely continue doing both every day or at the frequency that your dentist or periodontist suggests.

I am certainly not suggesting that you should stop brushing and flossing—just the opposite. Every time you go into the office for a professional cleaning, ask your hygienist to go over proper brushing and flossing techniques with you again. This will help remind you and keep you up to date on any new information regarding brushing and flossing. View your hygienist as your coach for gum care. A good coach can improve an athlete's performance in many ways. Ask a lot of questions and have them show you what to do each time you visit. Do not worry—if they are anything like the professionals I know, they will be delighted you are asking questions. It indicates that you care and that you "get it."

As a result, you could find yourself learning more information about caring for your gums than you ever dreamed existed. Your care provider should be delighted that you are talking about the subject they know so much about. You will find that most professionals will gladly share insights with you. This might also have the effect of them spending more time on your teeth because they know you actually care. Contrast that with the patient who just grudgingly sits there through the whole cleaning process and gets up and leaves without even saying thank you.

Remember that brushing should be done gently because it does not take a lot of scrubbing to break up plaque. We want to be careful not to erode our precious gum tissue while brushing. Once the anaerobic bacteria underneath are exposed to rich oxygen content, they will die or switch back to aerobic metabolism (some bacteria can do that). In either case, they will stop secreting the toxins that come from the anaerobic lifestyle. The word is *metabolism* for you sticklers out there!

To repeat from above, brushing too hard can erode your gum tissue. Obviously, that is something we want to avoid. In extreme cases, brushing too hard can expose root surfaces, remove too much enamel, and actually make your teeth more yellow-looking once you scrape away that surface enamel. Also, think about this: If gum tissue is diseased, it has to be weaker than healthy gum tissue. Therefore, it is even more vulnerable to recession from brushing too hard. Brush gently!

You might be wondering, just how hard is too hard? To illustrate the point that hard is not necessarily good, try a little experiment with me. This is going to sound silly, and you might even feel silly doing it. However, it might open your eyes to just how gentle you can be. Ready? Get out a pair of earplugs and put them in. If you do not have any, you can pick up a pair from your local drug store for just a few dollars. Once you have those plugs in, get out your toothbrush. After properly disinfecting your toothbrush, warm the brush under warm water. This makes the bristles a bit softer and gentler, as heard from our friend earlier. Turn off the faucet so the sound of the flowing water does not throw you off. Start brushing. With the earplugs in, you should distinctly hear, or feel, the vibration—I am not sure which is happening here—of those bristles against the teeth. When you hear that noise, see how gentle you can get. Using this technique, you should realize the right amount of gentleness you can use and still have the effect of cleaning plaque off your teeth. Again, double check with your dentist on proper brushing methods.

We want to save as much of our gum tissue as we can. We need it to help hold our teeth in place and to protect us to the greatest degree possible. If brushing too hard can cause recession, we definitely want to guard against brushing hard.

I mentioned above that you need to sanitize your toothbrush. There are various ways to do this. There are toothbrush sanitizers that use UV light to help kill the germs on the end of your toothbrush. You have worked hard to get germs out of your mouth, so there is no sense in putting them right back in when you brush next time.

Here is a link to a UV sanitizer: http://tobeinformed.com/sanitizer

If you do not have a fancy UV sanitizing device, just soak your brush in a little Listerine for thirty seconds.

If you need to make your teeth whiter, brushing harder is not the solution. Once your gums are healthy, you might consider whitening treatments or over-the-counter products for teeth whitening. However, teeth whitening products can actually burn your gum tissue. In addition, such products can be damaging to your enamel. There is no easy solution to teeth whitening. Later, you will learn about xylitol gum and a mouthwash cocktail that could help to lighten some of the stains on your teeth. Stains go hand-in-hand with plaque. If you have heavy staining on your teeth, then you probably have a fair amount of plaque buildup, as well.

I have heard some people say they like to brush with baking soda. One hygienist I spoke to said that it is too abrasive and could be harmful to your gum tissue. Yet, other professionals disagree and actually recommend using baking soda. Later in this chapter, you will find some information about baking soda that could make you think twice about using it.

If you really think you need to get the color of your teeth lightened, start with a professional cleaning to take off any surface level stains. Ask your dentist or periodontist for advice on whitening your teeth from there. There are many options available, and your health care professionals will certainly be happy to tell you about them.

As I mentioned before, despite what anyone says, using peroxide whitening products on your teeth *might* cause sub-clinical (not visibly noticeable) damage to your enamel. This can manifest as tooth sensitivity to liquids or sugary foods.

If the possible dangers mean nothing to you, if you are not interested in the expense of in-office treatments, and if you prefer to shop online, here are two options for tooth whitening products

that do not require any kind of prescription:
http://tobeinformed.com/wtsecrets (available in the US only)

http://tobeinformed.com/MTW (available internationally)

Most people brush absentmindedly and do not even realize how they are affecting their gum tissue. Interestingly enough, we often brush hard enough to erode the gum on the outside or the lip side of the teeth and not on the tongue side. Here is a little trick to help prevent that from happening:

> Brush the flats of your teeth first. What I mean by a "flat" is the top or bottom of the tooth, depending if it is a tooth on the upper side of the mouth or the lower side.

Next, brush the inside of the mouth, or the side of the teeth that faces the tongue. By the time you get to the outside or the lip side of the teeth, you will be thinking about what you are doing and, hopefully, brushing a bit more gently by that point. I learned this little sequence from a periodontist, so use it to your best advantage. Disregard this information if your own dentist does not agree with it.

Finally, we will talk about the amount of time you brush. Two minutes is the industry standard. That is the advice you are going to get from most professionals. Try using a stopwatch the next time you brush. You should be surprised to discover that you are not even coming close to two minutes. You might even find that you are only brushing for twenty seconds! That is a big difference and a huge gap in your oral health routine.

Here is an interesting article on how long most people brush:
http://tobeinformed.com/brushingtime

Flossing should also be a very gentle activity. There is no need to floss hard or jam the floss into your gums. The gums can suffer minor cuts that way and become sore and painful. If this happens, lay off flossing the sore area for a day. Wait too long and the plaque will build up. It is best to just be gentle from the beginning. No need to make a snapping sound when flossing either. Floss gently, because the plaque is not strong.

There is a difference between your gums being sore because of gum disease/gingivitis and inflammation from flossing too hard. If you are not sure which you are experiencing, ask your periodontist or hygienist to help you distinguish between the two. If you have gum disease and have not been flossing, pain is likely to be from the former and not the latter. Your gums should not feel pain from dental probing either. In a diseased state, they probably will. Trust me—you will know it when they probe your gums. If your gums are healthy, the probing will not bother you.

When the worst is over and you get control of your dental health, you might even like going to the dentist to get your teeth cleaned! The main reason is that you will not be feeling the pain you had been used to feeling.

The key to fighting or preventing gum disease is consistent, not hard, effort. This means that you remove plaque consistently on a daily or more frequent basis, depending on what your dentist recommends for you. Flossing once a week is not going to cut it for the same reason you cannot get away with brushing your teeth every other day without facing the consequences.

You can use up and down motions while flossing, or back and forth motions, or both. I verified this with my periodontist. I was wondering about this for a while and had read conflicting information about it. Being gentle is the key. The dental floss is meant to wrap around the tooth. I like to use ten to twenty up and down and/or back and forth motions. First one side of the tooth gets done, and then the other side. Repeat this process until finished. Be sure to learn proper flossing techniques from your dentist or hygienist.

Xylitol Gum

Xylitol gums, mints, and even mouthwashes are available in most health food stores. Xylitol is a five-carbon sugar, as opposed to a six-carbon sugar like sucrose (table sugar). Remember before when I said there were no magic bullets when it comes to fighting gum disease? That still holds true. However, xylitol can be a powerful ally in the prevention of cavities. Why? Xylitol is believed to work to fight the bacteria that cause dental diseases by providing them with a fuel they cannot use. Unlike sucrose, xylitol does not feed the bacteria in your mouth; it actually inhibits their growth. The little beasts cannot digest xylitol, despite their best efforts. They can literally starve to death on xylitol. Too bad for them! This gives your body's natural defenses time to rebuild the enamel in your teeth instead of being overwhelmed with toxins and acids produced by the bacteria. Xylitol is also helpful in fighting or preventing ear and sinus infections. In fact, xylitol is added to some nasal and sinus irrigation treatments exactly because of its bacteria-inhibiting abilities. By the same token, anaerobic bacteria that cannot process xylitol cause gum disease.

As humans, we have an alternate fuel-creating pathway that allows us to digest xylitol with no problem. There are a few people who cannot use xylitol for other reasons, but in such cases, xylitol is passed harmlessly from the body. Therefore, it does not hurt humans who use it, but those little critters we call bacteria cannot get energy from it. They try and they die. Plus, xylitol contains about a third less calories than regular sugar!

What is my personal experience with xylitol? It looks like xylitol chewing gum has helped to lift some of the stains that had accumulated around the exposed root areas of my teeth between office visits. It also leaves me with a nice clean feeling. I feel confident about chewing gum with xylitol because I know the bacteria cannot get any energy from it. I have found it to be a wonderful practice to rinse my mouth with water and then chew xylitol gum after a meal or snack, when it is not practical to brush and floss directly afterwards. It helps to normalize the pH of the mouth.

I am currently chewing up to twenty or twenty-five grams of xylitol per day. I like it and after reading quite a bit about it, I feel it is both safe and healthy to use. I am after the protective and preventive effects of the gum, so I will continue to chew it for the long term. There are also xylitol mints for folks who are already struggling with dentures and not able to chew gum.

There are tons of information and studies about xylitol that document its usefulness. In addition, there are decades of human experience with using xylitol—most notably in Finland. I could load you up with lots of references and studies and other boring information, but this is a layman's guide and most of us are not overly concerned about that kind of documentation. If you want to learn more about xylitol, including the evidence that supports its use and safety, head on over to www.xylitol.org. There is plenty of information there, and if you are a dentist or researcher, you can find many intriguing study references on that site, too. I should add that there are plenty of studies in the dental literature, as well.

When you first start adding xylitol to your diet, you should probably go a bit slowly in regards to the quantity of xylitol you use. Here is a funny story that happened to me. I was using both xylitol gum and mints freely, as well as using the powder form of xylitol to sweeten my drinking water—to get myself to consume more water. In high concentrations, and especially when you are just getting used to xylitol, you can get "the runs." Unfortunately, I went a little overboard on the xylitol mints and ate half a bottle in one day! That, in combination with the gum, and use of the powdered form in my drinking water, was a little too much. You can imagine what happened. To be fair to xylitol, there are people who regularly consume very large amounts of it daily, much larger than the amount I used, with no ill effects. Your body will get used to higher amounts, but watch out when you are first starting.

The good news about xylitol gets even better. Its use is good for diabetics because the breakdown of xylitol in the body to make energy is largely insulin independent—meaning it does not require the use of insulin the way glucose does. Diabetes is caused by a problem with the body's insulin production, and that problem is largely bypassed in the case of xylitol. It also appears that xylitol can help athletes achieve better performance. Last, but not least, xylitol can be useful in helping the body absorb more calcium from the gut while digesting food. This benefits those who are at a higher risk for developing osteoporosis.

Since this is a book about fighting gum disease, we shall get back to that topic. Several studies have been conducted that strongly suggest through statistically significant results that chewing xylitol gum can reduce the incidence of dental cavities. Since the same kind of bacteria are believed to be responsible for gum disease, using xylitol gum could be useful in fighting or preventing gum disease, as well. At the very least, it will not feed the bacteria in your mouth the way sucrose will. I have also read that xylitol might actually lift dental plaque from the teeth, making it easier to brush away. This could prove to be a powerful tool to help fight the development and/or progression of gum disease, as well as help prevent cavities in the first place.

In addition, studies indicate that the daily use of a certain amount of xylitol gum may be enough, over a period of time, to create a protective effect against dental caries. An interesting study showed that even after months of no longer chewing the gum, the study group seemed to continue enjoying the cavity-preventive effects of xylitol. This could very well be due to a shift in the type of bacteria that inhabit the mouth after long-term use of xylitol. This protective effect lasted years after one particular study ended, even though the participants stopped chewing the gum. This is powerful. It has been suggested from studies that these benefits might be derived from chewing about six to ten grams of xylitol in gum form per day for about six months or so.

I believe that most dentists are aware of what xylitol can do and the numerous studies associated with it. Xylitol and its effects have been known for many decades. Has your dentist mentioned xylitol gum to you? Not one of the many dentists I have had an office visit with over the course of my entire life, so far, has ever told me about xylitol gum and its protective powers.

Not all xylitol products are created equal. Some of them contain another sugar alcohol called sorbitol. While sorbitol gum has also been shown to reduce the incidence of cavities over glucose (regular sugar) gum during studies, they did not achieve the same results as xylitol.

One possible reason for this is that while those bacteria cannot use xylitol at all, they can use sorbitol in a reduced fashion. Those bacteria have trouble using sorbitol, meaning they cannot use it as efficiently as glucose, but some bacteria can still use sorbitol for fuel in a limited way. Therefore, my personal opinion and inclination would be to avoid even sorbitol gum in favor of gum sweetened a hundred percent by xylitol. In other words, I do not want to see sorbitol mixed in with xylitol in the ingredients of any xylitol product I wish to use. The same holds true for malitol and other glucose alternatives as well. Malitol and sorbitol are six-carbon sugar alcohols, similar to glucose. Xylitol is a five-carbon sugar that appears to confuse the bacteria—they think they can eat it, but they cannot.

Xylitol has been widely used in Finland since WWII. The dentists there noticed the effect it had on patients' dental health, and they have been using it ever since. A hygienist told me she took a trip to Finland, and found that the Finnish are so proud of xylitol in their products that the word "xylitol" appears in inch-high letters on their packaging. It has worked well for them for decades. So why do we not use it?

The effects of xylitol have been well documented in professional literature. If a dentist told me that he/she had never heard of xylitol before, I would be hard-pressed to believe it. There is plentiful information available about xylitol. Yet, as mentioned previously, I was never told about xylitol by any of the dental professionals I have visited. Hopefully, that will change in the future.

It is amazing to me that we have not replaced our glucose-laden foods with xylitol. Obviously; doing so would be so much healthier for our entire society.

WARNING: While xylitol is safe for human consumption, it could be harmful to animals. Do not feed xylitol to your pets!

You can find xylitol gums and mints, as well as the powdered form of xylitol, in most health food stores. If you would like to purchase xylitol products online, you can visit this address: http://tobeinformed.com/xylitol

Mouthwash Cocktail

A dentist, Dr. Ellie Phillips spoke to me in absolutely glowing terms about a combination of very common mouthwashes you can find in practically any drug store. She has experimented with all kinds of mouthwashes and has yet to come across anything that comes close to what these three—in her opinion—can do.

Dr. Phillips, or Ellie, as her friends like to call her, has written special directions for the proper use of these three mouthwashes, and she is very adamant that users follow these directions, too. Fortunately, they are published on her website at this location—http://tobeinformed.com/epmouthwash. The directions are part of a document called *Zellies Complete Mouth Care System.*

When I heard about this mouthwash cocktail, I decided to give it a good try. I followed her directions and I can honestly say that this combination made my teeth very smooth and clean feeling. The mouthwash combination is made up of three mouthwashes that you are probably already familiar with. The three are Listerine, CLÖSYS and ACT.

Be sure to read Dr. Ellie's directions. Again, she mentioned that she has experimented with all kinds of mouthwashes and this combination is by far the best, in her opinion. Get permission from your dentist to try this out for about two weeks and see if you notice a the difference, too. I am more than willing to bet you will.

The ACT mouthwash contains fluoride, and you will be using it frequently in Dr. Ellie's system. This brings us to an area of controversy: fluoride.

She does offer a slight variation in her directions if you want to avoid the use of the fluoride. But, that fluoride rinse can harden your enamel is widely accepted as true. From questioning her, I found that she is rather adamant about the use of the fluoride rinse and that the replacement she suggests in her directions may not be as effective.

From what I understand, the fluoride rinse will actually react with the natural minerals that are in your saliva and cause your teeth to harden. In addition, the reaction with fluoride forms a 'crystal' that is 'more perfect' and harder than what your teeth would be with the same minerals sans the fluoride. This makes your teeth smoother and offers even less places for bacteria and dental plaque to adhere to. That's one theory. There is at least one chemist, named Gerard Judd, who talks about the use of fluoride having a negative effect on both teeth and gums.

As I probably mentioned before, I am not that interested in taking sides on the fluoride debate. Besides, this is a book about fighting dental disease and cavities, and what we are most concerned with is what works to achieve this. Even though I am not taking sides, I felt compelled to ask Dr. Ellie about the use of fluoride in her system then give you at least one voice from the other side of the fluoride debate. First, let me share my question and Dr. Ellie's response with you.

Ellie,
If the fluoride atoms are ending up in your teeth, then the next time you ate or drank something acidic that breaks down the enamel, wouldn't you end up ingesting those fluoride atoms as well? David

Dr. Ellie's Response:

Dear David,

If you are worried about this amount of fluoride—you should definitely stop drinking tea (up to 8 ppm) eating yams (12 ppm) and consuming a laundry list of many other products that either naturally contain fluoride or are contaminated with it.

*In the perfect world I would agree this **might** be something to think about.*

I am practical by nature, and (as with most things) I believe it is a question of balance.

If you have no risk of mouth acidity or dental problems, perhaps you do not need the added protection of fluoride.

If you have nature, age, harmful bacteria, or dietary problems working against you, I would recommend the fluoride rinse to protect yourself from dental fillings and help smooth teeth to avoid plaque depositing.

I would rather accept a minuscule and debatable risk than have a white or silver filling, and the associated harm, stress (very damaging to the body), and other possible side effects!

This mindset that is "knee-jerk" to the word fluoride is precisely why many "holistic" consumers walk around with horrendous teeth; they avoid all fluoride (they think) but end up with worse problems from the treatments they ultimately require. I'll accept this possible and small—maybe even non-existent risk! [Doctor's Name Removed] is always very outspoken about fluoride, yet talks of plaque on his teeth and the need for fillings and dental work...

It is great to live in a country of choice. I would never tell people they have to accept my views; I would urge them to see things in balance. Good question—but I think we need to look at the proportion of risk to benefit!   *Ellie*

      ❖   ❖   ❖

Dr. Ellie brings up some good points. Smoothing the teeth so that they are less sticky for plaque and bacteria to adhere to certainly sounds to me like it would help in preventing cavities and gum disease!

To be fair, I feel that I must present someone's argument from the other side of the fence.

This link is a short read. This Internet page about fluoride was written by an MD and quickly summarizes the basic arguments that you will hear from those who staunchly oppose fluoride and the reasons why:

         http://tobeinformed.com/fluoride-danger

Dr. Ellie does not carry the pro-fluoride battle alone. Here is a link to a fluoride proponent site:

         http://tobeinformed.com/fluoride-info

In case you were wondering—PPM means Parts Per Million.In the case of a food having 8-PPM fluoride, that basically means that if you broke that food down to a million little parts, 8 of those parts would be fluoride.

What about my own personal results with Dr. Ellie's directions? Here is what I can tell you: I only had a chance to use her sequence for about two weeks before my last dental cleaning.

During that time, I watched stains on my teeth, which were already starting to lift from chewing xylitol gum, reduce even further. I have never seen my teeth as white and clean as after that last dental cleaning. Whether this was due to the xylitol gum or to Ellie's formula or both, I cannot say for sure because I started using the gum perhaps one or two weeks before the formula. In any case, I was delighted by these results.

I have found that using the Hydro Floss before following Dr. Ellie's directions is very beneficial as it removes the larger food particles from the mouth. This gets them out of the way so that following her sequence is not inhibited.

Once again, Dr. Ellie's directions can be found here:

http://tobeinformed.com/epmouthwash

The Perio-Aid

I have seen additional improvement of my gum tissue when I added a Perio-Aid to my routine. One hygienist commented that a Perio-Aid can really help to firm up gum tissue. I have found this to be true. This is because it stimulates the tissue and can have the effect of making it stronger.

It was the Hydro Floss that initially helped my gums to stop bleeding, but the Perio-Aid really added to the results I achieved. This is a valuable tool for your gum health, so do not underestimate it.

Here is what a dental hygienist who visited my site had to say when she saw that I mentioned the Perio-Aid:

Hi Dave...I just read your post and it looks great! I had to laugh when I read that you also use the Perio-Aid. I love the Perio-Aid, too!

How about Stimudents from Johnson & Johnson? They are a tried and true tool that have been around for probably more then 50 years. They are great for interdental stimulation and toughening of the gums. They are also a very handy tool to keep with you on the go! I always recommend keeping them in the car or pocket to have them handy. (Forgive me if this is also a tool mentioned in one of your writings that I have not read.)

For people who have not yet started with professional care, Stimudents have been recommended to "test" for periodontal disease or gingivitis. When used with slight pressure between the teeth to massage the gums, if the person sees bleeding at all, there is infection and it needs to be dealt with.

If only gingivitis, it may heal with improved home care alone, but if there is deeper damage (Periodontitis) the person really needs the professional assessment and treatment to clean out from under the gums, and then all the good tools for daily home, and 2-3 month professional cleanings to help keep the destruction from periodontal disease under control. As you recommended, professional treatment should always be sought.

It is better understood now that there is a relationship between gum infection and general systemic health problems, but we also comprehend much more of the two-way relationship of gum disease and risk for diabetes and pre-term low birth weight babies and for heart disease and stroke. It is very telling that some of the insurance companies will now pay for periodontal treatment for pregnant women and diabetics as they are realizing that it is more cost effective to help with the gum disease than pay for the complications that arise with systemic health issues where gum disease has been an added factor in the lifetime costs of caring for the complications that arise with a pre-term low birth weight baby or the health problems of the diabetic.

I hope I have not gone on and on too much on this issue, but it is a passion of mine that people understand the link and the importance of oral health. I am not a researcher or lecturer, but a clinician who loves to explain and instruct my patients in what they can do to make a difference. Hey, if they work harder, my job is easier too! It makes dental cleaning visits more comfortable if patients take responsibility for their daily routine, and of course, the tooth decay and other dental concerns become less and less, too. It all works together for keeping patients healthier and happier in every way. Thanks again for a forum to hear me out.

All the best and continued success in getting the word out that people can help themselves to better oral and systemic health by taking time in their own daily routine!

Hillary, RDH, BSDH
Holland, PA

✲ ✲ ✲

The Perio-Aid is a device that has curves on the handles and a clamp-like mechanism that is used to hold part of a toothpick on each side. The ends are labeled with the numbers 1 and 2. The two ends are used in different parts of the mouth. It is easy to keep it straight if you can just remember this: the side labeled 1 is for one area only—the bottom six teeth on the inside or tongue side of your mouth (also called the lingual side). The side labeled 2 is for everywhere else.

I have to admit that I have gotten different stories on how to use the Perio-Aid from different hygienists. Another hygienist told me that it does not matter which side you use for any given part of your mouth; just use what works best for you. Be sure to ask your periodontist or hygienist to explain the best way for you to use the Perio-Aid.

The Perio-Aid is used to trace along the gum line primarily. It gets the little "u" shaped area, or sulcus, of each tooth. These are spots that flossing might not adequately reach. Anywhere the dental plaque is not disrupted provides protection, a home, and acts as a breeding ground for those nasty anaerobic bacteria that harm the health of our gum tissue and tooth enamel. Remember to remove that plaque daily. The Perio-Aid helps you to do that. The Perio-Aid has the added benefit of stimulating the gum tissue to help it become healthier.

Do not underestimate the power or the value of a Perio-Aid. Remember that many dental professionals really like this tool. However, it is entirely possible that you never heard of it before. My previous dentist never told me about it. Yet, if you have gingivitis or gum disease, you really ought to know about it.

The Perio-Aid was actually created by a periodontist. I love it when solutions come from within the industry. It adds relevance and credibility. Sometimes, the person with the most expertise comes up with amazingly simple but powerful solutions. The Perio-Aid qualifies as an amazing device that is easy to use. Get one, if you do not already have it.

Once you get instructions from your hygienist or periodontist on the use of the Perio-Aid, you will find that it is convenient and easy to carry it in a pocket or a purse. This is one of the nice features of this tool. I often carry mine in my laptop case or even in my pocket.

I have heard that some people use it while watching TV. Of course, I do not recommend that you use it while walking or otherwise engaged in any activity that requires your full attention, such as driving a car. You could hurt yourself—or even worse, you could hurt others. Do not take any chances where safety is concerned. It is not worth it. Just use it at home when you are not moving around. Using it while looking in the mirror will most likely give you the greatest level of control.

The Perio-Aid is an important tool, but I have not seen it sold in any drug store I have visited. To get one you will have to ask your periodontist, and they usually give them out freely. I cannot imagine that your periodontist's office would not have them. If they do not, drop by another periodontist's office and request one.

Here is a web page that has pictures and simple directions for using the Perio-Aid. The link was valid at the time of this writing:
http://tobeinformed.com/perioinstruction

The Hydro Floss

The Hydro Floss is a type of oral irrigator. Oral irrigators have been around for quite some time. The Hydro Floss itself has been around since the early 1990s.

The Hydro Floss is my favorite tool because it did a lot of the work towards getting my gums healthy. Do you remember my story from earlier when my dentist wanted me to sign a document stating that it was not their fault if I lost my teeth? The Hydro Floss is what I used to escape having the SRP treatment that my dentist recommended. I cannot guarantee it will do the same for you. I can only tell you that it worked in my case.

Opinions vary among professionals regarding oral irrigation. You can talk to some who really like oral irrigation and others who are lukewarm (or even cold) about it. However, studies have proven the Hydro Floss's ability to reduce tartar (calculus) and plaque buildup between office visits. Is that valuable? If you have read sequentially up to here, you already know that it is.

Here is another interesting letter from our hygienist friend in Pennsylvania in which she mentions oral irrigation:

Hi David,

Just wanted to say hello.

I am a Dental Hygienist who has been in practice for over 33 years.

I want to commend you on your information. It is great and I hope it reaches out to many, many people.

I am a very good hygienist, both as far as my clinical skills and communication skills, but I know very well that the answer to people keeping their gum disease under control is really, mostly in their own hands.

It is the daily commitment to oral care that will make the difference in the long run. Of course the tools used are critical and I wanted to just let you know that I am a huge fan of oral irrigation!

You are so right in your letters. I can only reach those who come to me in practice, but you are doing a great service to people who will not or CANNOT go to a dental office.

Just wanted to compliment you on the work you are doing.

All the best,
Hillary, RDH, BSDH
Holland, PA

My Reply:
Hi Hillary,

Thank you so much for your kind note. I really appreciate what you wrote and let me say that it helps me to carry on when I get notes like this one. So thank you again.

I definitely am a fan of professional care. I've worked hard to make sure people know that the first thing they should do is see a periodontist and get regular dental cleanings. I even use my own example of two-month intervals for professional cleanings.

There really is no substitute for professional care.

Yet, as you mentioned, what people do in between visits is extremely important. Not much can be done in the long run if people ignore their home care or do a poor job of it.

As you are well aware, it is very possible to keep your natural teeth healthy for a lifetime. But, so many people won't be able to do that simply because they don't understand the basic facts.

Let's continue to help them understand the truth about gum health.

Hillary, Thank you so much again.
Warm Regards, David Snape

※　※　※

I am currently aware of two studies that have been done specifically on the Hydro Floss oral irrigator. One study was done in 1993 on the effectiveness of the Hydro Floss that uses magnets to polarize the minerals in water in order to do a better job of reducing the accumulation of plaque and tartar from your teeth and around your gums. To my knowledge, the Hydro Floss is the only oral irrigator that utilizes this technology.

The second study was done in 1998. Both indicate or at least suggest the effectiveness of the Hydro Floss. Of the two studies, the former appears to yield the most conclusive evidence. In the interest of making sure my information is accurate, I bought a copy of one of the periodical journal articles for my own review. It was on the study completed in 1993.

Here is what I posted on one of my websites in regards to this study:

Since I've taken to the habit of quoting a study done on the use of magnetic devices in conjunction with oral irrigation, I thought I better make sure I didn't misquote or misstate anything.

Therefore, today I purchased a copy of a study published in the May 1993 issue of the Journal of Clinical Periodontology. I purchased my copy from the Blackwell-Synergy website.

The title of the study is The Effect of Oral Irrigation with a Magnetic Water Treatment Device on Plaque and Calculus. *(ISSN 0303-6979)*

Quote from the study: "The measurements of the group using an irrigator with a magnetic device showed a 44% greater reduction in calculus volume (p<.0005) and a 42% greater reduction in area (p<.0001) over the group using an unmagnetized irrigator."

Of course, they don't mention in the text of the study what magnetized irrigator they used, however it is revealed within the study.

On page 2 of the published article which is page 315 of the Journal issue mentioned above, there is a diagram. At the top of the diagram it is clearly printed: Hydro Floss Research Project.

The study seems to validate what the experience of myself and others has already shown us: The Hydro Floss works!

Here is what I can tell you about the Hydro Floss for sure: It stopped my gums from bleeding! I am not a dental professional, but I do know that at one point, blood was coming from my gums during my regular dental cleanings. I used the Hydro Floss and the bleeding stopped. When I went back to the hygienist, they said my gums looked much better and that I did not need that root scaling and planing treatment after all. That is the bottom line for me. The Hydro Floss saved me time, money, and pain. I still use it every day.

Currently, I use the Hydro Floss to shoot a jet of water at right angles to the gum line (not 45-degree angles). This is another point where I have found varying opinions among professionals. There does not seem to be universal agreement about whether you should use the Hydro Floss water stream angled at a 45-degree or a 90-degree angle. The argument against the 45-degree angle is that you may push the tartar further down under the gums. I am not sure if that is a valid argument or not.

When I first started to use the Hydro Floss, I would shoot the water at a 45-degree angle and straight down into the gum line. However, when I went to a periodontist's office, the hygienist told me not to do it that way. She also told me to put the Hydro Floss on a lower setting. She said that you should be able to squirt the water stream directly under your tongue without feeling any pain. That is how she believes you can gauge the correct setting of an oral irrigator for yourself. She also said to angle the stream of water at a 90-degree angle, not a 45.

The Hydro Floss Company seems to indicate that even the highest setting will not harm gum tissue. My personal feeling is that it is best to err on the side of caution. You can always move up, so start on a lower setting.

Now, bear in mind that it was when I was shooting the water stream at a 45-degree angle, my gums quit bleeding. I do not offer you any advice on this at all, except that you should ask your dentist or periodontist about this and follow his or her advice and instructions regardless of anything you read here. I am only telling you what worked for me. In addition to using the Hydro Floss, I also added a few capfuls of an oxygenated mouthwash to the Hydro Floss reservoir so that the mouthwash would be delivered directly to my gums. You will read more about that mouthwash soon and what I replaced it with, next.

I discovered that it was simpler and more convenient to use something called AktivOxigen Serum instead of the oxygenated mouthwash. You simply put eight drops in the Hydro Floss reservoir before use. The bottle is very small because it is concentrated. The small bottle is much more convenient to use compared to storing and accessing bulky 16-ounce bottles of mouthwash.

Another great use of the Hydro Floss is to rinse the teeth after eating a meal and before brushing. It gets a lot of the larger food particles out to increase the effectiveness of brushing, flossing, or otherwise clearing the mouth of debris.

Do not get bogged down with the different options expressed here because the Hydro Floss comes with directions for care and use. For some reason, the instructional video that normally comes with the Hydro Floss was not included in mine. I wrote to the manufacturer, and they sent me the video at no cost to me.

If for some reason the instructional video on using the Hydro Floss does not come with yours, you can use the link below to view the instructional video online. If you are thinking about the Hydro Floss for yourself, this video can also be very informative.

http://tobeinformed.com/vidhydro

If you want your own Hydro Floss, you can get one at the following web address and get free shipping by using coupon code **A-PER10**: http://tobeinformed.com/hydrofloss. A free bottle of the AktivOxigen Serum also comes with the Hydro Floss when ordered from the above link. The benefit to using this AktivOxigen Serum with your Hydro Floss is that oxygen can kill the anaerobic bacteria by interrupting their cellular processes.

You can see a picture and read about the AktivOxigen Serum here:

http://tobeinformed.com/oxygen-serum

The Hydro Floss also comes with four tips—one for each family member. This is a great way to introduce children to superior oral health home care at an early age.

Since I have experienced the power of the Hydro Floss firsthand, I would like to share my experiences with you. Here are two articles from the past that I have written about the Hydro Floss:

The Hydro Floss Oral Irrigator Worked for Me

Why do dental professionals tell us that up to eighty percent of adults suffer from some form of gum disease? I feel like I have been misinformed in regards to what it takes to get rid of gum disease or prevent it in the first place. Gum disease is a serious problem. It can cause a person to lose some or all of his or her teeth. Yet, so many people walk around oblivious to the fact that they have gum disease.

Many dental professionals do tell their patients how to fight or prevent gum disease. For some reason, sometimes there can be found a dental professional who does not teach his or her patients about what they can do to stop or prevent gum disease.

Occasionally, that same professional could be prepared to provide expensive treatments when things get really bad. That age old saying, "An ounce of prevention is worth a pound of cure," seems so apropos in regards to gum disease.

When my hygienist and dentist wanted to perform a procedure called a scaling and root planing on me is when I began to take serious notice of the problems my gums were having. Up until then, I did not really think that I had gum disease.

I did not like the sound of the procedure they described to me and decided to do some research to find out if there was anything that could improve my condition without having to go through the treatment. One of the earliest and most effective things I tried was the Hydro Floss oral irrigator.

My results were so good with this instrument that the next time I visited the dentist they actually told me that I no longer needed that root scaling and planing treatment and that there was no longer any tartar buildup under the gum line. To me, that was exceptional. I could also tell by the look on their faces that they were a bit surprised, too.

After a lot of follow-up investigation, I realized that sometimes the professionals do not always know best. For example, when I initially told my dentist that I wanted to get a Hydro Floss, she said that they were too expensive and that I should buy another, less expensive, oral irrigator instead.

I did not listen and I bought a Hydro Floss anyway. I am glad I did. I would buy another one tomorrow if something happened to mine. It is sturdy and rugged and really holds up. I do not know if other brands of irrigators could hold up as well.

It constantly amazes me when seemingly unaware dentists attack the way the Hydro Floss is alleged to work. The theory involves something called hydromagnetics. I have heard and read about dentists who say this is all bunk, there is absolutely nothing to this technology, and that it provides no additional benefit over regular irrigation.

Some of them argue that it is impossible to polarize (put a charge on) water molecules. What they do not realize is that the charge is placed on minerals in the water, not the water molecules themselves. The Hydro Floss Company, somewhere in their literature, tells you to use tap water. This is precisely because there are minerals in tap water. If you used pure distilled water, there would be no minerals to polarize.

It causes me some mild concern to know that those dentists probably have not read their own profession's literature. A study was published in the Journal of Clinical Periodontology in May 1993 suggesting that oral irrigators that use hydromagnetics do a superior job of tartar reduction over non-hydromagnetic irrigators. The differences noted appear to be statistically significant. There is only one oral irrigator I have found that utilizes hydromagnetics and that is the Hydro Floss.

If you have, or think you might have, gum disease or any other oral health problem, visit your periodontist or dentist for advice, diagnosis, and treatment. This article is for information purposes only.

Hydro Floss Review—It Works!
I have had my Hydro Floss for at least two years now and I can tell you that it has been a huge help to the health of my gums. My gums used to bleed during dental cleanings. My hygienist and dentist eventually recommended that I have what is called a scaling and

root planing treatment to remove tartar that had built up under the gum line.

Upon further questioning, I decided that I did not like the idea of a scaling and root planing treatment, so I declined. I was also a little perplexed. I was not really told much about gum disease by my dentist, although I was told I needed this treatment in a hurry. Were there not any preventive measures that could have been taken years ago? I was disappointed in my care provider.

I went home and started looking for a solution. I tried a few different things but I did not see much improvement. Finally, I came across the Hydro Floss. I called my dentist and she actually told me NOT to get one. She said I could just get another oral irrigator and it would be just as good, but would cost less. She said she did not believe in the claims of the effectiveness of the hydromagnetics that the Hydro Floss uses.

When I got off the phone, I knew I was going to get one. I lost faith in my dentist a long time ago and if she said it was not good, then it probably was good. (Ah, the strange logic there!) Turns out, I did the right thing.

When I returned for my next exam and cleaning, I was actually told that I no longer needed a scaling and root planing treatment. The hygienist said there was no longer any tartar under the gum line. She even said there was no bleeding while probing. I was told to "keep it up." They acted as if I had been following their directions all along.

Why should I have to be the one to figure out what works for gum health? They should have been the people to tell me what to do to fix my gum problems.

4827rte

I wrote a book entitled, *What You Should Know about Gum Disease* in order to share my experiences with others. My frustration with the lack of information about gum disease made me realize that other people could use the information I have found and utilized. In addition, I discovered other products that worked for me besides the Hydro Floss and I have added them to my book, as well.

As far as my dentist not believing in the power of the Hydro Floss, I have something to say. This isn't a matter of believing or not believing. Perhaps she doesn't keep up with her profession's literature. The Hydro Floss is mentioned in a study published in the Journal of Clinical Periodontology. This study showed how much more effective the use of the Hydro Floss with a magnet was versus an irrigator that did not use a magnet.

I don't know if your dentist is anything like mine. But, I have learned a valuable lesson. If you have or think you might have problems with your gums, visit a periodontist. They have additional training and experience with gum disease. Periodontists are dentists with two years of extra training. Their focus is on the health of your gums.

Reader Experience:
Day Four on the Hydro Floss

HOWDY Dave,

I am still using my Hydro Floss.

I still have red mad gums, however I think it might be helping the bleeding. They seem to not bleed as much, it is not an instant fix along with my hard work of consistent brushing and flossing and such. I think in time this just might be the key.

84

I used it 2 times yesterday; it does not hurt. The first day it seemed to make my gums more mad but I wonder if this is the healing process? I go in for a cleaning by the Dentist the 9th of next month so we'll see from now till then if we can conquer this deal!

More tomorrow!

Heather

My Reply:

Hi Heather,

This is great news. I am so happy to hear of your initial success and am looking forward to hearing more.

This is very similar to my own experience with the Hydro Floss. I watched as my gums became better over a period of a few months with the Hydro Floss.

When I went back to the dentist a few months later, they were visibly amazed, though they didn't say anything. It was kind of like they didn't want to acknowledge the Hydro Floss.

My dentist just said, "keep doing whatever you are doing," as if she didn't know I was using the Hydro Floss.

Keep up the good work.

Dave

❅ ❅ ❅

Ordering the Hydro Floss by Telephone
It is not surprising to hear from folks who prefer to order by telephone. Here is a request I received from a man who wished to purchase the Hydro Floss by telephone, followed by my response:

*I will only order Hydro Floss by phone, not online; kindly forward #
to call, or call me at* [number removed for privacy]. *—Thanks, Ed*

My response:

Hi Ed,

Here is the number to call:

Call 1-800-97-FRESH

Ext. 2296

*Tell them you want to use coupon code A-PER10 to get free
shipping.*

M-F 8am-5pm PST (California Time)

❖ ❖ ❖

Essential Oils
The next tool that I have used, but am not currently using, is an
essential oil blend. It is a mixture of three oils: peppermint,
spearmint, and almond. The blend comes in a small bottle with a
drip-proof top. It takes about one or two drops mixed with your
saliva to produce a very biting taste and a saliva/oil mixture that is
alleged to kill the bacteria that causes bad breath and gum disease.
(The FDA has not evaluated such claims.)

There is a very long-standing mouthwash on the market today that
is accepted by the ADA (American Dental Association). If I said the
name you would recognize it instantly. Since this mouthwash contains a large amount of alcohol, it would be easy to presume that the
alcohol was killing the germs. I am sure it contributes, but taking a
close look at the active ingredients gives us another clue. You will
find eucalyptol, thymol, and menthol on the label. Those ingredients

are there for a reason. Now, it is not such a far stretch to see how essential oils might be able to kill bacteria, right?

If you use the oil blend three times a day, a single bottle will last about three months. In that sense, it is a pretty good deal. This product is available around the world, and they offer free shipping.

Remember when we talked about balancing pH earlier? After using this essential oil blend you definitely will want to do something to shift the pH closer to neutral again. Use a mild pH mouthwash as a follow-up and chew xylitol gum. At the very least, thoroughly rinse the mouth with clean water.

I used to carry a bottle of essential oil blend around with me for use after each meal. It can be used with or without a toothbrush. The leak-proof top actually works. I never had one drip or leak, and I carried it extensively.

If I ate a meal and did not have access to regular toothpaste and a toothbrush, I would often use this essential oil blend, instead. You can follow the easy and simple instructions on the bottle. Be prepared—it has a strong taste!

As far as its effectiveness goes, I cannot accurately gauge that. It was the use of a Hydro Floss that caused my gums to stop bleeding. I used this formula about the same time or slightly before.

There is a website where this product is sold with a large number of testimonials from happy customers. You can find more information about this essential oil blend at: http://tobeinformed.com/oils

I am not currently using this product, even though I have tried it in the past, because there are plenty of other tools and products in this book I am currently using. However, I still thought it was a good idea to include it here because there are probably some folks living in remote places around the world who would not have ready access to a drugstore. The company that makes this product will ship it to virtually anywhere in the world that has mail service.

Every person's body is different and what worked for one person will not necessarily work for another. So I do not have reservations about mentioning the oil here. I have noticed the website of a dental hygienist with many years of experience and she talks about this product in a positive way.

When I phoned in an order to the company, the person taking the order said that this essential oil blend got her gums to stop bleeding in about two weeks. It did not do so for me, but everyone is different.

One of my concerns about this product is that even though it is potentially helpful, I am leery about the idea that it can work *all by itself* to eliminate gum disease. My understanding about gum disease tells me that the mechanical removal of dental plaque is crucial to conquering gum disease. Brushing, flossing, use of the Hydro Floss, the Perio-Aid, and similar such devices can manually disrupt the plaque, which is an important step towards conquering gum disease. However, this essential oil blend could be helpful in conjunction with the mechanical removal of plaque. It certainly does not hurt to reduce the harmful bacteria population in your mouth.

You can read some customer testimonials about this product here:
                    http://tobeinformed.com/oiltest

Mouthwash

Another tool I have used is an oxygenated mouthwash. I actually used to add this compound to the Hydro Floss's reservoir before using the Hydro Floss to clean around the gums. Once I discovered the AktivOxigen Serum, I found it a lot easier to work with. The mouthwash is called PerioTherapy Oral Rinse. This is a mild pH mouthwash. I like to call it a friendly mouthwash!

You can find it at this web address:
http://tobeinformed.com/perio-rinse.

Once again, the AktivOxigen Serum can be found here:
http://tobeinformed.com/oxygen-serum

PerioTherapy Oral Rinse is for helping to combat gingivitis and gum disease. This formula uses the PeriO2 compound. This is a very special formula made of stabilized oxygen compounds. The oxygen is useful in killing anaerobic bacteria. That would include the bacteria that cause bad breath as well as the bacteria that cause gingivitis and gum disease.

I found this mouthwash to be very soothing to the gums. It contains Aloe Vera as well. I rate this formula highly as I do the other similar formulas I have used from the same company. PerioTherapy mouthwash has a mild pH. You can find more information on this rinse at: http://tobeinformed.com/perio-rinse

Theoretically speaking, the use of the oxygenated compound should have a negative impact on the anaerobic bacteria because they cannot thrive in the presence of oxygen. Put too much in their environment and they either die or switch back to aerobic metabolism. Either outcome is a victory for you.

PerioTherapy mouthwash and toothpaste can sometimes be

found at local stores. You can read more about them here:
http://tobeinformed.com/details

Toothpaste and Gum Care Kit
PerioTherapy toothpaste uses the same oxygenated compound as the mouthwash previously mentioned. In addition, it contains Aloe Vera, pyrophosphates, zinc gluconate, and ubiquinone. Ubiquinone is also known as Co Enzyme Q-10, which you have possibly heard of. Both the mouthwash and the toothpaste are available together in a product called the complete gum care kit.

You can read about the toothpaste at:
http://tobeinformed.com/perio-toothpaste

You can read about the complete gum care kit at:
http://www.tobeinformed.com/gum-care

The gum care kit comes with moldable trays that allow you to keep the toothpaste in contact with your gums a bit longer. In addition, it contains the oxygenated mouth rinse. The gum care kit also comes with some very special gum disease fighting tips that I think are worth reading. I would reproduce them here, but they were written by Dr. Katz of the California Breath Clinics. He is a dentist who has devoted his life to creating sensible products for combating bad breath, and he has also formulated products for helping in the fight against gum disease. You can get a free copy of his book, *The Bad Breath Bible*, at this address:
http://tobeinformed.com/bbbook/

You can also get the PerioTherapy starter booklet free from this site: http://tobeinformed.com/periostarter

There are two things about this toothpaste that some could see as detractors. The first is that it contains fluoride. Fluoride is useful for dental health because it hardens the tooth enamel and protects us against cavities. However, as mentioned earlier, some are adamantly opposed to the use of fluoride even in toothpaste and mouth rinses. I am well aware of the debate that rages on against the fluoridation of our drinking water. As I previously stated, I am not interested in taking sides on the debate at this time. I am less concerned about the fluoride in toothpaste and mouth rinses because they can be spit out before being ingested. There are drawbacks to everything and it just is not possible to cover all the bases.

There are a lot of studies, thoughts, and ideas about the use of fluoride; it is a hot topic in many circles. I prefer not to get involved in the raging debate right now as I do not know where the various factions will eventually find common ground. However, if you are dead set against the use of fluoride in your toothpaste, then this toothpaste obviously would not appeal to you. I wanted you to know what is in it so that you can make a choice based on your personal preferences.

The second detractor is that the toothpaste contains sorbitol, as do many other toothpastes. While it is true that sorbitol has been shown to reduce the incidence of cavities in studies, there is another facet to using sorbitol that should be considered, one that we discussed earlier. The bacteria in our mouth cannot use sorbitol the same way they use glucose. However, some bacteria can break down sorbitol for energy, although the amount of energy they can extract is greatly reduced. A better choice, if you have to sweeten toothpaste at all, would be to use xylitol.

There are toothpastes available that contain xylitol, though you might have to hunt a bit to find one. Usually, they are not sweetened a hundred percent with xylitol and have mixtures of sorbitol, malitol, or other sweeteners. Check out your local health food store if this is the direction you choose.

In today's world, where we eat a lot of refined sugars and drink a lot of enamel-damaging colas, we need all the advantages we can get to protect the health of our tooth enamel and our gums. PerioTherapy toothpaste is a good choice overall, despite the potential detractors to some.

The following is from a reader of my site (edited):

Hi Dave,

Thank you very much for your invaluable information about gum disease.

As I said before, using some of your products has made a huge difference to my gums; my teeth look whiter, gums are pink and less puffy and there has been no more bleeding at all...and of course my breath is fresher even in the morning.

I use my mouthwash after lunch at work and I floss morning and evening. Unfortunately I still enjoy my coffee and red wine but I try to rinse my mouth every time I have something that could stain my teeth. God, I'm becoming obsessional!

I have been using Hydro Floss with AktiveOxygen, the PerioTherapy toothpaste and mouthwash as well as the OraMD oil, which I use after hydro flossing.

I have also been experimenting with 10% iodine solution and grape seed extract solution and the results are really great especially since the GSE has a broad antibiotic role.

I do have a dentist phobia and I have not contacted a periodon-

tist. However I am lucky as one of my best friends is a dentist and she has been regularly removing plaque off my teeth (only over the last 2 years).

I think my gum problems are moderate in severity and mainly confined to my maxillary where I inherited my father's crowded teeth. I am conscious that I have to see a periodontist and I'm ashamed to say that I have not got the guts yet.

Name Withheld

❊ ❊ ❊

Though there are a number of other tools that I have tried and will probably still use from time to time, I think that diligent use of the Perio-Aid, Hydro Floss, oxygenated mouthwash (or AktivOxigen Serum) along with gentle brushing and flossing are important parts of my arsenal for good home care. Chewing xylitol gum and use of the mouthwash cocktail have become part of my regimen, since this email conversation occurred, as well.

Electric Toothbrush

My opinion differs from others regarding electric toothbrushes. Although they have been shown to reduce plaque more effectively than regular toothbrushes, I believe using a regular toothbrush properly can be quite effective. To be fair, studies do tend to suggest that the electric version works much better.

Electric toothbrushes generally require the replacement of special and relatively expensive "heads" or brushes. In addition, I believe you can be gentler with a regular toothbrush because you have greater control. I prefer a regular brush because I want to be as gentle as possible when brushing.

I do have an electric toothbrush, and I have tired of replacing the head and keeping the battery charged. In addition, it is a lot easier to travel with a regular toothbrush than to bring your electric along with its cumbersome charger.

Besides, I also have regular floss, the Hydro Floss, the Perio-Aid, and other items to help fight gum disease. However, if you have an electric toothbrush and feel you are getting good results, by all means, continue using it! Remember that the ultimate goal is to remove troublesome plaque on a regular basis. Every effective weapon that helps you fight and prevent dental disease is worth its weight in gold.

There are several different kinds of electric toothbrushes. Some of them have timers on them. Timers are useful because most people do not brush their teeth for the minimum two minutes that they should. In fact, many people brush less than twenty seconds. This means it is very likely that many spots are missed, and plaque is not being removed as well as it should. With the timer, you will be surprised at how little time you spent brushing previously.

I have been to several different dentists over the years, and they all have their own preference and recommendations. I will not mention what kind of electric toothbrush I use, because you should go with the recommendation of your periodontist if you choose to utilize one.

Again, if an electric toothbrush gets you to brush longer or brush in the first place, then it would certainly be worth it to have one. An electric toothbrush can be one more weapon in your arsenal of tools for fighting gum disease.

If you would really like to have an electronic toothbrush and must shop online, you can find a premium one here: http://tobeinformed.com/electric-brush.

I do think it is best to follow the recommendation of your periodontist, however.

Scaling and Picking

It is unlikely that your dentist has told you about scaling and picking. Even though the tools are available at many drugstores, you should ask your dentist if it would be advantageous for you to use them. You should also ask your dentist or periodontist for specific instructions. Do not use these tools without your dentist's approval and instructions.

If your experience has been anything like mine, then you have likely noticed a peculiar circumstance after getting your teeth professionally cleaned. At first, whenever I had my teeth cleaned, they would be whiter looking but within a week, I would notice stains developing again.

Obviously, it is not practical to get your teeth professionally cleaned once per week. Even my two-month schedule appears excessive to most people. What is one to do when the stains build up so fast? If you walk into a major drug store, such as CVS, you will find scalers and picks for sale. They often come with special blue lights attached to them, or the lights might be on a mirror that comes with them, to increase visibility—or you might not find a light at all. There are different brands that have their own specific features. You can use these instruments to remove stains that start to build up on your teeth. Basically, the professional cleanings done in dental offices employ tools similar to these.

If you get the nod from your dental professional, you should give it a try and see if you are able to reduce the stains that accumulate between professional cleanings. If you are able to do that, you could find your teeth remaining a little whiter for a little longer between professional cleanings.

I am always amazed to watch the pick or scaler remove stains right off the surface of my teeth. If you use a hand-held mirror when using these instruments, you will see exactly what I mean.

When finished with picking and/or scaling, be sure to rinse the mouth out. You could have dislodged clumps of bacteria and plaque and there is no need to swallow those. Instead, rinse the mouth out and get them outside of the body where they will trouble you no longer. Scaling and picking is something I would consider doing about once or twice a week, in addition to, not instead of, other regular home care. I personally have not seen the need to use these on my own teeth lately. I do not often use them. Yet, it is something you can discuss with your dentist if you think it would benefit you. One thing is fairly certain: Your dentist probably has not told you about the availability of these tools.

Regular Flossing

Flossing is a necessary and useful method of helping you remove plaque. It is something that you should be doing on a daily basis.

Unfortunately, too many people actually do brush and floss regularly, but still develop gum disease. In my opinion, if brushing and flossing were enough, we would not be seeing the high incidence of gum disease that professionals encounter.

If you are not fortunate enough to be among the twenty percent of people who do not have some form of gum disease, maybe you could get by with only brushing and flossing. If you are like me and the other eighty percent of adults out there, you need more than just brushing and flossing to help maintain your gum health between office visits.

We discussed flossing in a bit more detail earlier in the book. I mention it again here as a reminder that you should be doing it. It is best to learn proper flossing techniques from your dentist or hygienist in person. They can coach you and check your technique in real time. Plus, they will be happy to see you wanting to learn. If you are not already flossing, you should be. I prefer dental tape over dental floss.

Using Salt Water as a Mouth Rinse

I hesitate to put this information in here, but I have found this to be a useful practice. Once again, do not do it unless your dentist gives you approval. If you have high blood pressure, are on a sodium-restricted diet, or have any other health conditions, you also need to check with your physician before doing this. Some of the salt will be absorbed into your body no matter how well you flush your mouth after using salt water. Therefore, you need to seek a stamp of approval from both your dentist and your doctor.

What I do is simply put some salt into water and make it moderately strong. I have never measured the exact amount I put in, but I can tell you that the salt does not completely dissolve. Therefore, as you get closer to the bottom of the glass, you will get a higher concentration of salt water. I take a mouthful and swish it around for about twenty to thirty seconds. Then, I spit it out and take another mouthful and repeat until the cup is empty.

Why do I do use salt water? There are two reasons. One is that the salt will stimulate your saliva, which can be useful in both eliminating bacteria and in protecting your tooth enamel. The second reason is that bacterial cells are a little bit different than human cells. There is a term known as osmotic pressure in physi-ology. Without getting too technical, the bacterial cell membranes can be ruptured, effectively killing the bacterium (single bacteria) when it is exposed to high concentrations of salt outside of its cell membrane.

Human cells, also known as eukaryotic cells, are a bit more resist-ant to the presence of salt. Once again, I caution you to check with both your regular doctor and dentist before attempting to do this. If they say no, then do not do it. I only know that it has been a successful practice for me.

Using Sodium Bicarbonate (Baking Soda)
Some of the hygienists I have talked to about the use of baking soda do not like the idea. Yet others do. *I have stopped using baking soda in my mouth altogether because of the information you are about to read.*

I happened to have a conversation with a dentist who has several decades of clinical experience. I have altered my views of baking soda as a result, and I am staying away from it for the time being. Here is part of our conversation:

Hi Dave,

Yes, it is very weird why this happens - I think that after about three times the gum tissues become sensitized to baking soda. I can't prove it and there is obviously no research that I know of. Baking soda is alkaline so you would expect it to be good - I don't know why it is not. I would suggest you might do a small sample test - maybe you could go to your local health food store one day. Ask the employees and possibly their customers (if the owners agree) who has used baking soda and/ or peroxide on their teeth.

Question number two would be if they have gum recession.

It might be interesting!

Just an idea - Anyone I talk with who has unexplained recession is positive every time.

Let me know if you find out more.

Name Withheld

❊ ❊ ❊

This dentist has had loads of clinical experience, and if this is a trend that she has noticed, I do not doubt the validity of the information. Still, without a lot of other supporting evidence, it is difficult to prove conclusively. You probably know my philosophy by now—it's better to err on the side of caution. Therefore, I have decided to curtail my use of baking soda. You will, of course, need to make your own decisions with the input of your own dentist.

To put some perspective on it, there are no studies that validate this notion about baking soda to be true. But that does not mean it is not true. The experiences of this dentist with the people she has worked with would be called anecdotal evidence. When an overwhelming body of anecdotal evidence exists, the hope would be that some researchers would come along and put together a study to validate or invalidate the theory. Unfortunately, that has not happened yet.

Research requires funding. Usually, companies will fund research on items when they can foresee a return on their investment. Which company or government agency would be willing to provide funds for a study about baking soda?

So you will have to draw your own conclusions on all of this, of course.

Sodium Ascorbate and Calcium Ascorbate

These both come in a crystalline powder form available at health food stores. I have added these because I have experienced what subjectively appears to be an interesting effect from using sodium ascorbate. I imagine that calcium ascorbate would be even better due to calcium's ability to help harden tooth enamel via our saliva.

I have only used sodium ascorbate so far. The effect I have noticed is that my gum tissue actually became what I can only describe as thicker. I say this is subjective because it is a perception on my part. I have used no instruments to measure progress and I did not record any type of baseline before I started. No study that I am aware of has been done on this, either. Since this is a book about my experiences and I have decided that sodium ascorbate has been helpful to me, I have added this information.

Sodium and calcium ascorbate are both forms of vitamin C. We do not want to use ascorbic acid because it is an acid. It is also rumored to not be as easily absorbed into the body as sodium or calcium ascorbate.

Once again, I caution you not to do what I did, but rather to check with your dentist or periodontist to see if this is something they are comfortable with allowing you to do. What I did while testing this out for myself was take one or two teaspoons of sodium ascorbate in a bit less than a cup of water and use it as a mouth rinse. I did this at the very end of any cleaning routine I was using on my teeth and gums. I would actually swallow this rinse because it is simply vitamin C, and I reason that it is good for my body. I would use this rinse two or three times a day—after cleaning routines.

Within about two or three weeks I noticed what I believe to be a thickening effect on the gum tissue. To give proper credit, I obtained this idea from a book by Gerard Judd, a professor of chemistry whose opinion on fluoride I briefly mentioned earlier. His book is titled: *Good Teeth, Birth to Death.*

I make no definite claim about using this rinse whatsoever. I can only tell you what I believe the effect to be on my gum tissue. As with everything else in this book, you should check with your dentist before attempting to make or use this rinse.

Sample Routine for Home Care

You might be wondering, "How do I put all this together?" What I am going to share with you is a sample routine. It is not my normal routine, as I like to mix it up a bit and improvise as I go. Yet it can serve as an outline and it might be useful to have a quick sample list to learn from. Again, check with your dentist or periodontist before doing any of this; if they say no, then do not do it. It could interfere with their treatment plan. If, for some reason, you are not sure about any particular doctor's advice, you always have the option of seeking second or even third opinions from other dentists, periodontists, or oral surgeons.

One routine is to simply use Dr. Ellie's mouthwash cocktail. Again, directions can be found at: http://tobeinformed.com/epdirections

Another option would be to follow a routine like this:

1. Clear the larger particles out of your mouth with a quick

pass of the Hydro Floss. Another oral irrigator could be used as well, but remember that the Hydro Floss has been shown to be more effective at reducing plaque and tartar buildup over irrigators that do not use the same technology.

2. Next, use a mouthwash that will alkalize your mouth. Perhaps the CLÖSYS mouthwash would be a good choice; it is what Dr. Ellie starts with in her system. She has told me that it is very useful towards clearing up pockets. You could also consider any of Dr. Katz's mouthwashes: http://tobeinformed.com/mouthwash. They all have a mild pH.

3. After using an alkalizing mouthwash, brush the teeth gently, using the sequence outlined earlier. Be sure to use brushing techniques approved by your dentist and hygienist. You might use either the PerioTherapy tooth-paste or another toothpaste of your personal choice.

4. Floss gently using the techniques taught to you by your hygienist or dentist. I prefer ten to twenty up-down and/or back-forth movements for each side of the tooth. The better you can wrap the floss around your teeth, the more surface area you will get. At no time should you cut into the gum tissue. The tissue will naturally resist and you will feel that natural barrier at the point where the tissue is firmly attached around the tooth. Go no further than that. Again, gentleness is the key. No need to do anything hard or quick.

5. Use the Perio-Aid according to the techniques taught by your dentist and hygienist.

6. Place eight drops of the AktivOxigen serum into the

Hydro Floss reservoir and fill to the top line with tap water. Use the Hydro Floss according to the instructions that come with it, or according to your dentists or hygienist's instructions. When I first started out, I used the Hydro Floss several times a day. Remember that I was on a mission to avoid that SRP treatment back then!

7. Use an alkalizing mouth rinse again. Remember that we want that final pH to be higher.

8. Finally, use the homemade sodium ascorbate or calcium ascorbate rinse as previously described.

Again, this is a sequence I *might* use on any given day. As I mentioned before, I like to mix things up a bit. I do not follow the same procedure day in and day out. I wanted you to have an example of my routine for your own reference. I believe it is important to alkalize the mouth before brushing in any case.

Chew xylitol gum or use xylitol mints between meals and snacks. After a snack or meal, I like to rinse my mouth first to rid the mouth of larger food particles. If no toothbrush is available, then I simply chew the xylitol gum. Its protective effect is something that, in my opinion, anyone with gum health problems or even dental cavity problems should definitely be interested in applying to their own situation.

Aside from chewing xylitol gum after snacks or meals, a routine like this could be done two or three times per day, or at the rate your dental care provider suggests. In addition, one might brush, floss, and use a mouthwash after meals. If you follow a routine such as this twice a day, or at the rate your provider recommends, plus use xylitol gum or mints between meals, it is hard to imagine you would not see improvement in your gum health by your next office visit. However, each person is different. Therefore, you could find it necessary to do even more than what is listed in this simple outline. It is also possible that you need less. In any case, only do what is approved by your dentist or periodontist. Do not take any chances with your gum health or the health of your teeth.

As a recap: Home care and professional care work hand-in-hand to help you prevent or fight gum disease. To maximize your effectiveness at fighting or preventing gum disease, you really need to utilize both types of care. Remember that dental plaque needs to be removed every day for the rest of your life. Consistency, not brute force, is the key to better home care.

You should ask your dentist or periodontist about these tools before using any of them. Make sure that their use does not conflict with the treatment plan your periodontist, dentist, or oral surgeon has recommended for you. You should follow the instructions of dental care professionals above all and seek their approval before attempting to use anything in this book.

*It is only when we forget
all our learning
that we begin to know.* —Henry David Thoreau

Questions about Gum Disease

I HAVE A blog that accepts questions, and this chapter contains some of the questions people have asked me. Many of my answers have been modified from the originals for the purposes of this book. If you are interested in asking your own questions about any health, fitness, or wellness topic, including gum disease, you can do so here:

http://tobeinformed.com/ask-dave-a-question/

✳ ✳ ✳

Can I Have Veneers or Lumineers if I Have Gum Disease?

Question:
Since I've been following your advice my gums look much better and I am thrilled about it.

I'd like to know whether in the future, if things improve, I could have any dental work such as veneers or Lumineers etc. perhaps gum grafting?

Many thanks. [Name Withheld]

My Reply:

Thank you for the feedback. I'm really happy to know that others have found my information and shared experiences helpful. Of course, I'm careful to tell others that I'm not providing advice because that is the realm of doctors and dentists. Instead, I tell others about my experiences and share some of my thoughts about gum disease.

Can you have veneers or Lumineers? Since your gums are getting healthier that is a very good sign. Once your periodontist feels that your gums have been restored to an optimal health level perhaps you can have veneers or Lumineers installed. That is a question that your periodontist, dentist, or other specialist will be able to help you answer. If he or she does not do such work, you can most likely get referred to someone who can.

I've done a bit of looking around and have found that there are patients who are not satisfied with their veneers. I've read where one person never felt comfortable with them and couldn't get their professional to make corrections after a certain point. This is a problem, because veneers are expensive.

Lumineers are much thinner and cost about seventy-five percent what porcelain veneers cost. Though sometimes there are problems with them that can lead to tooth decay or even gum disease. So be very careful, do your research carefully, and find someone who is really good to install them.

To avoid problems, you may want to take some steps to protect your investment. Choose your professional wisely in the first place. My best suggestion is to first get references and then try to figure out who may be the most precise, thorough, and caring in their practice.

Then, interview several professionals during the 'initial consultation.' Ask a lot of questions and watch how they respond. If they get agitated or show the slightest degree of frustration over your questions or aren't willing to spend extra time with you, that might be a warning sign. You want someone who puts the care of their patients above the bottom line numbers of the business. That may take some looking.

It is really important to choose a professional that you like and feel comfortable with. If you have an uneasy feeling about any professional, find another one that you do like. It is hard to follow the advice of a professional that we don't fully trust. You also want to feel comfortable that this person will be there for you if problems develop and you need extra care or more care than the average patient to make things right. You don't want to be caught in a situation where you spent a lot of money for mediocre or less than ideal results and have no way to get things corrected without spending even more money.

Again, ask lots of questions—any professional who won't patiently answer your questions, whatever they may be, should probably be abandoned in favor of one who will. Check and double check the information he or she provides you. This is how you can intelligently build your confidence and trust in a health care provider.

Don't be in a hurry. Develop a thorough understanding of what you are going to be receiving and possible problems that may arise. Ask your professional of choice how they would respond to such problems if they should occur. Above all, be willing to walk away if you are left with any nagging question marks. I'd rather spend a little time and find someone who will do the job right and that I'm comfortable with than find myself stuck with a big bill and unsatisfactory results.

I prefer the look of natural teeth over any covering. However, everyone is different and situations are different. Getting veneers or Lumineers may very well be the right choice, depending on your personal situation.

I Have a Gum Tissue Pocket - How Do I Get Rid of It?

Question:
I have an open pocket near the molar. I also start to get a very painful sensation whenever I floss the area. I think it's due to gingivitis. But honestly, I really don't know how it came about. Which leads to my general questions: How did this happen? How do I get rid of it? Is there any way to prevent it from happening again?

My Reply:
Hi and thank you for asking these questions.

You probably do have gingivitis or gum disease. You'll need your dentist or periodontist to confirm. I've noticed that oftentimes, people think their gum disease is localized to a specific area. Yet, people are surprised when they go in for an appointment to discover that their whole mouth is having a problem.

Aside from the pain, does it bleed when you brush or floss? Gum disease can be present whether there is bleeding or not. There should NOT be any noticeable pockets around any of your teeth. In fact, the pocketing that occurs in mild gum disease shouldn't be noticeable to the eye.

What you should do first and foremost is solicit the aid of a good periodontist. He or she can assess the true situation in regards to your gum health. Unfortunately, the layperson may not be able to tell how extensive his gum disease is. You believe it only affects this one area. However, there is a good chance that your whole mouth has been affected. Go to a periodontist and get your situation checked out immediately.

How did it happen?

It's not unusual at all and more people have some form of gum disease than you might imagine. It happens all of the time. Anaerobic bacteria living under a thin biofilm called plaque are the cause of gum disease and cavities. If you have a lot of plaque buildup, your teeth and gum tissue could be under constant attack from the acids secreted by bacteria. This can cause both cavities and gum disease.

Gum disease is a problem that can start at any time in life. I believe that in most cases it starts early and grows slowly worse over time. Most people have no idea how to tell reddish diseased gums from pink healthy gum tissue. It sounds like it would be easy to tell just by looking, but it is not always that easy. You really need to have put in some study and have the practical clinical experience in order to tell the difference, or be trained in what to look for. In addition, probing for pocket depth and tissue loss as well as x-rays may be needed for the diagnosis. A dentist or periodontist should examine you as soon as possible. They can give you an actual diagnosis and recommendations.

How do you get rid of it?

First, visit your periodontist and carefully consider his or her recommendations. Obviously, I can't tell you what type of problem(s) you are facing, but I can tell you that going to a periodontist will be worth the investiture of your time. The periodontist will give you his or her recommendation and you can choose what to do from there. You may also want to ask your periodontist what type of things you can do at home in addition to regular brushing and flossing to help alleviate this problem and stop it from returning. Battling gum disease is a continual lifetime commitment. Maintaining dental health requires varying degrees of work at home, in addition to professional care, depending on a person's individual conditions.

How do you keep it from coming back?

Your periodontist or dentist can help you develop a home treatment plan to be followed in addition to your regular cleanings and check-ups. You may want to partner with your dentist and ask him if it is okay to incorporate some other tools into your home care plan.

The mouthwash cocktail, Hydro Floss, and Perio-Aid are three tools you should consider asking your periodontist about. If they give you the green light, these things are likely to have a powerful effect on your dental health. [See Chapter 3]

Unfortunately, most of us just don't know how to fight gum disease or prevent its occurrence in the first place. And, it seems that worthwhile information is not widely available or just poorly understood. If you start working on this now, you may be able to solve your problem and prevent any similar ones from arising again. Fighting or preventing gum disease is a lifetime battle.

❊ ❊ ❊

Can Gum Tissue Grow Back?

Question:
Can gum tissue grow back after receding?

My Reply:
Yes, gum tissue can grow back, but the amount that can grow back may be limited. If you keep the area meticulously free of plaque and tartar you may see some regrowth of gum tissue that was previously lost.

Surgery may also help with the replacement of tissue under certain conditions. Results, however, may not be optimal. Gum graft surgery or bone matrix insertion can help in this regard to some degree. Again, the results may not be ideal with these two proce-dures.

There is a gel called Emdogain that may be used in conjunction with gum surgery to help regrow gum tissue. It came onto the market back in 1997. It can be injected during surgery and has been shown to achieve good results. You can ask your periodontist if Emdogain can help you or not.

Your best bet is to do everything you can to prevent recession in the first place or prevent your current recession from getting any worse. As time goes by, technology may find even better solutions. For now, your best bet is avoiding that recession in the first place.

If you are reading this, take a lesson from our experiences. Stop recession from happening in the first place. If it is too late for that, then work to stop it from getting worse! Our mouths are the largest gateway to the external environment. Is it any wonder that they can get so dirty and build up so much bacteria that cause us problems? Getting your dental health back and maintaining it from here on out are both very important.

Thanks for asking your question. If you have any others, please do feel free to ask them at:

http://ToBeInformed.com/ask-dave-a-question

❊   ❊   ❊

Are Teeth Whitening Products Safe When You Have Gum Disease?

Question:
I'd like to know if it is safe to use teeth brightening products if you suffer from gum disease.

My Reply:
Thank you for asking this question. It is one that I have wondered about, too. Short answer: I wouldn't try it until your gum tissue is completely healthy again.

First, let's talk about the effects of tooth whitening on enamel, and then we will move to the gum tissue. I did a little search on the Internet and found a site that says tooth whitening does not damage enamel. Of course, they were selling a tooth-whitening product. Unfortunately, I have found contrary information from legitimate studies.

You can reference PMID: 17437883 (PMID= Pub Med ID). In this paper, you can find the description of micro changes that occur to the tooth enamel from carbamide peroxide bleaching agents of both sixteen and ten percent.

Carbamide peroxide is the bleaching agent that comes in most home whitening treatments. Even doses stronger than ten percent exist and they can often be found in dental offices for in-office bleaching procedures. They may also be sold in various retail stores such as your local drug store.

In-office procedures may also use hydrogen peroxide concentrations of up to thirty-eight percent. Another pub med listed study (PMID: 17432790) showed a loss of calcium from teeth treated with thirty-eight percent and thirty-five percent hydrogen peroxide (with light) over the control group. However, they did not find statistically significant calcium loss from the users of ten percent carbamide peroxide over the control group.

The article, PMID: 17380806, showed nano and micro changes in the enamel in short term and long term bleaching respectively. The layer of enamel was found to be reduced by the bleaching procedures.

On the other hand, the study documented in PMID: 17339072 showed that there were no problems found in enamel hardness or in any other areas studied in relation to the use of hydrogen peroxide bleaching strips.

Now as for the gums, I did not find any references on the effects of bleaching agents on gum tissue. However, and this is just my opinion, if gum tissue is diseased, it is probably weaker than healthy gum tissue. Being so weakened, it may not be a good idea to expose it to any chemicals that could cause further damage.

Personally, I would prefer to 'Err on the side of caution,' as the saying goes. Consider seeing your periodontist for a professional opinion about tooth whitening and what type may be best.

Anything chemical that is strong enough to make your teeth whiter might have a harsh effect on the gum tissue. Why not work on getting those gums back to a healthy pink condition before considering any type of whitening?

Some products and techniques might have the effect of making your teeth whiter as plaque is reduced. This happened to me both with the use of xylitol gum and the 'mouthwash cocktail.' [See Chapter 3]

Thanks for asking your question and giving me an opportunity to answer it.

❖ ❖ ❖

Bad News from the Dentist

Question:
Dave, I just came from the dentist's office today and they gave me some very inturbidating options. They said I have Stage Four peri-

odontal disease and want to pull all of my top teeth as I qualify for a grant that would buy dentures.

Any type of surgery etc. for me is iffy, as I have low blood clotters, which may be saving me from things like high blood pressure, etc. and which may be the result of my taking herbs.

However, I told the person helping me that I know of two people who turned their gum disease around. You are one of them.

My question is, yours is probably NOT as advanced as this, Stage Four, right?

Although they don't think so, I know ALL things are possible. The "experts" said that the world was flat, that airplanes wouldn't fly, that cancer, polio and arthritis are incurable. The experts were wrong.

So knowledge is power and putting works to faith is what I best be about (like using my Hydro Floss machine, which I haven't yet, o-oh, but will tonight!)

I've got to keep my spirit up. And so God is assisting me in doing that.

Anyway, just thought to communicate and ask you what you did.

Take Care and keep up the good works.

My Reply:
Hi, and thank you for asking this question.

My first impulse is to tell you to go get a second, and perhaps, a third opinion. Some doctors may have greater experience and knowledge than others. This is a case where you do not want to act rashly. It sounds like you have time to research, get opinions, and make a more informed decision. I personally would not agree to having my teeth pulled on the advice of a single office.

I was not anywhere near "stage four," but I did have problems.

I also am not completely out of danger. I will need to be on guard and diligent for the rest of my life, as should the majority of people be. I have to prevent gum disease from creeping back and that means diligently removing and preventing the formation of plaque. For me, that entails a bit more work than just brushing and flossing, as it does for most people.

I assume that by using the term "stage four" that your dentist means the most advanced form of gum disease. My case of gum disease was still in the early stages, but beyond mild gingivitis. Because my lower front teeth are crowding, I had trouble keeping plaque buildup off the back of them. That is one of my danger areas.

Though I may not lose my teeth, I have to be diligent in cleaning my teeth and gums every day.

What is important about gum disease is keeping the plaque from building up, and it builds daily. So, there is a combination of things I did and continue to do.

As you know, the Hydro Floss solved my bleeding gum problem. Yet, I found that though my pockets seem to be reducing from the use of the Hydro Floss, it didn't eliminate them completely by itself. Of course, you must brush and floss. I use the Perio-Aid. The mouthwash cocktail [mentioned in Chapter 3] seems to have accelerated improvement even further. In addition, it gives my mouth a nice clean feeling. I'm brushing very gently without bending the bristles too much. I'm flossing with regular dental floss. In addition, I get my teeth cleaned every two months. I've found that I build stains and plaque very quickly, and getting a professional to clean them more frequently has proved to be invaluable. With the addition of xylitol gum and the mouthwash cocktail, I have a feeling that the rate of plaque and stain buildup will reduce even further.

If you look in your mouth, you can sometimes see the areas where plaque and stains have accumulated. I think the stains and plaque go hand-in-hand—where there is one, you will often find the other.

Your situation sounds difficult. It makes me wonder: Now that they can get a grant, they are willing to do this? Have things really changed that much since your last 5 visits? Again, I'm thinking you should get a second opinion and even third opinion before getting all of your front teeth pulled. Have you been to a periodontist? If you are not sure about getting your teeth pulled and wonder if they can be saved, it might be worth your time to visit other doctors to see what they have to say. I'd be cautious about taking the advice of an office that can get a grant to do this kind of work on you— without more opinions.

❄ ❄ ❄

Gum Disease, Cavities, and Fluoridation

Question:
Hi Dave,

I am interested in fluoride and gum disease. I have heard that fluoride makes no difference to gum disease and that about 50% of all teeth that are lost are lost due to tooth decay. Do you know about this and can you confirm it? Thanks, if you can assist.

My Reply:
Thank you for your question. Let me attempt to answer the tooth loss question first.

In the course of my ongoing investigation into gum disease and how to get rid of it, I have come upon many statistics. Sometimes, the statistics seem to contradict each other. However, the majority point to gum disease as the number one cause of tooth loss.

One dentist explained that there is a high percentage of tooth loss due to cavities before the age of twenty-five. After that, the majority of tooth loss cases are due to gum disease. If you think about it, you can get a cavity filled, so it should not cause tooth loss very often unless it is not taken care of.

Regardless of whether a person loses a tooth due to gum disease or tooth decay, the underlying problem is exactly the same. Bacteria, and the plaque and calculus they live in, cause both tooth decay and gum disease. Bacteria live in our mouths and use our mouths as their bathroom. Those toxins and acid secretions accumulate on the teeth and around the gums.

When plaque forms, the bacteria have a nice home in which to live and multiply rapidly. Then a larger amount of toxins are produced, which can more rapidly cause both tooth decay and gum disease. So whether you are trying to prevent cavities or gum disease, the cause is widely agreed upon to be the same: the anaerobic bacteria that live under the plaque.

To answer your question on fluoride: Official government sources still say that certain levels of fluoride in the water are useful for preventing cavities. There are individuals out there who say this is not true and that fluoridation is harmful to the body in many ways. I'm not taking sides on this issue at the moment.

As far as fluoride helping to prevent gum disease, here is what I can tell you: My periodontist has his hygienists use fluoride during cleanings. I asked about this and they said that even though there is a debate, they believe it is useful in fighting gum disease.

There is a chemist named Gerard Judd. He talks about fluoride possibly destroying a key enzyme that binds gum tissue to the tooth. I do not know that any studies have been done on this. I'm just telling you that there is someone out there who makes such a claim.

I hope this covered your question thoroughly enough. If not, you can simply ask another question at:

http://tobeinformed.com/ask-dave-a-question/

Please remember that this is for information only. If you have or think you might have gum disease, a cavity, or any other oral health conditions, contact your dentist for diagnosis and treatment. Thank you for submitting your question!

❋ ❋ ❋

Where Can I Find OxyD-8 Oral Care Products?

Question:
I couldn't find OxyD-8 on Google. Any suggestions?

[In case you are wondering what prompted this question, I have a video on YouTube.com about the Hydro Floss. You can watch this video.

I'm not an expert at video so if it looks a bit amateurish, it really is. However, it is the content that matters. Here is the link to the video: http://tobeinformed.com/ytvideo]

My Reply:
Here is a link to the PerioTherapy mouthwash, which is different than the OxyD-8 formula mentioned in the video: http://tobeinformed.com/perio-rinse

[**Note:** This site information has been changed from the original formula in the video because I believe that the PerioTherapy Oral Rinse is a more appropriate formula for the purpose of helping to fight gum disease rather than the one shown in the video. It uses a compound similar to OxyD-8. The OxyD-8 is used primarily in fighting bad breath. Both release oxygen to kill anaerobic bacteria.]

Online, a bottle will cost you around $14, but you can sometimes find this mouthwash in a drug store. They might sell it at your local Wal-Mart or Target too. Offline, you can usually get it for around $9 for a nice savings.

The other option is to buy in bulk online where you can obtain a really nice savings, even when compared to the lower cost of buying individually in retail stores:

http://tobeinformed.com/gum-health-formula

This bulk package includes several tubes of toothpaste, as well.

* * *

Bad Breath and Its Causes

Question:
What causes bad breath, and what is the best way to stop it?

My Reply:
Aside from some really obscure and dangerous conditions and dis-

eases of which bad breath is a side effect, there isn't a whole lot of official, government-sponsored information out there on situational, or even chronic, bad breath. I was hard pressed to find much worthwhile information about "regular" bad breath from such sources.

These government sources said things like: brush your teeth and tongue, use a fluoride toothpaste, floss, and don't smoke. Also, there was some mention of using fresh parsley or a strong mint to temporarily freshen the breath.

One thing they did mention was that many mouthwashes do not treat the underlying problem. That's for sure!

All of the above is generally good (and obvious) advice, but if any of that worked for everyone on more than a temporary basis, there would be very little bad breath to suffer in the world.

And, we know that isn't the case, don't we? In fact, a lot of people suffer with bad breath.

Many mouthwash companies target bad breath directly and they wouldn't be doing that if there wasn't a market for it.

Don't think that it has to do with how well you take care of your mouth. For most people, that is not the case. You can brush and floss all day long, but if you do nothing to get at the root of the problem, those things won't help much beyond their temporary effects. It is not a question of impeccable oral hygiene, although that can definitely help.

Unfortunately, many of the products for sale may not be all that good for fighting or stopping bad breath. They tend to mask the bad breath temporarily. Some could possibly make it worse after their initial effect wears off. For example, some products may have a drying effect on the mucous membranes inside the mouth.

Since official documentation was quite lacking, the best information I could find on bad breath was from Dr. Harold Katz.

He offers a free forty-seven-page e-book on bad breath. If you don't mind leaving him your email address, you can get the latest copy here: http://tobeinformed.com/bbbook

Doctor Katz says that bad breath is due to anaerobic (can't live well with oxygen around) bacteria that live in the folds of the tongue, back of the throat, and in between the papillae of the tongue. These are areas that don't normally get exposed to much oxygen.

He also says or implies that these little critters naturally exist in your mouth and you won't be able to completely get rid of them. However, when they multiply out of control, they produce volatile sulfur compounds (VSCs) that are responsible for foul smelling breath.

Things like smoking, coffee, alcohol, dry mouth, snoring, and mouth breathing are all factors that can make bad breath worse. Regular toothpastes that contain sodium lauryl sulfates (soap) can dry out the mouth tissues, contributing to more bad breath. Dr. Katz has specially formulated products that don't contain SLS or alcohol.

Saliva naturally contains oxygen which works to keep the little critters or anaerobic bacteria down to a minimum. However, if the mouth dries, there is less oxygen around. With less oxygen, the bacteria thrive more. With more bacteria, there will be more volatile sulfur compounds hanging out.

When the VSC levels reach a certain point, you will have noticeable *bad breath. Drinks like coffee and fruit juices increase the acidity of the mouth, which also causes the anaerobes to reproduce more quickly. They like a more acidic environment. Of course, sugar helps them as well.* [Bad breath is an additional reason to pay attention to the section on pH presented earlier.]

You asked what the solution was. Download Doctor Katz's book at http://tobeinformed.com/bbbook and I think you will find the answers you are looking for.

If you have bought any of about eighty-five percent of the bad breath solutions on the commercial market including mints, breath sprays, and mouthwashes, you have ended up disappointed or with very temporary results. Breath mints don't work for very long, nor do they get to the root cause of the problem.

I trust Dr. Katz—and if I were trying to get rid of bad breath, I would use Dr. Katz's stuff. I'm not certain that there is much else out there that will work as well without undesirable side effects or short term results.

Here is the link to a free trial that will give you a chance to sample Doctor Katz's products for bad breath:
http://tobeinformed.com/trial
There is a $6.95 shipping and handling charge at the time of this writing.

* * *

Why Do My Gums Bleed When I Floss?

Question:
I don't like flossing because it makes my gums bleed. I know a lot of other people with the same problem. Can you suggest a way to stop it?

My Reply:
It is not normal to see blood while brushing or flossing your teeth. A person with bleeding gums should see his dentist as soon as possible.

Bleeding gums are most likely due to gingivitis, or, its big brother, periodontal disease. These are both unhealthy conditions of the gingiva or gum tissue, it is just that periodontal disease has progressed further than mere gingivitis.

I used a Hydro Floss Oral Irrigator daily to get my gums to stop bleeding. Of course, there are no guarantees that the Hydro Floss will work for you because everyone is different and comes from a different situation. One thing is for sure, the Hydro Floss stopped my gums from bleeding.

Periodontal disease is more advanced than mere gingivitis. Both need attention to help prevent tooth loss and other potential health problems. Gum disease usually begins with bacterial growth inside a biofilm called plaque. The gums become irritated, which causes them to bleed and separate from around the tooth, forming a pocket. A person suffering from gum disease could lose the supporting structure around the tooth (including bone) and, finally, the tooth itself.

The situation doesn't need to progress that far and there are things you can do to improve your dental health. The daily mechanical removal of the plaque is important to prevent gum disease or to stop its progression. You also should be working with a periodontist or dentist to receive a diagnosis and recommended treatment plan. He or she can help you to review all of your options.

You may know some people who have lost many or even most of their teeth. To prevent experiencing a similar situation, it is impor-

tant for a person to pay close attention to the state of his or her gum health.

Bleeding of the gums is also dangerous in that once there is a breach in your gum tissue, where bleeding occurs, it is possible for bacteria to enter your blood stream and further infect the body.

In order to stop your gums from bleeding, there are two things you need to have in place. Professional care is one, and excellent home care is the other. One alone will not solve your problem—you need both.

By the way, you are definitely not alone in having gums that bleed when you floss or brush. Things can get much worse. Get help from a dentist or periodontist; pick one you really feel comfortable with.

An Anonymous Comment Left On One Of My Blogs:
When I wake up in the morning my teeth will already be bleeding. It has gotten so bad that I don't even kiss my husband, and I explained to him why I don't.

I brush my teeth every day, and while brushing them they will bleed, so I at least have to brush them 3 times back to back, then I gargle my mouth with mouthwash, and it will stop the bleeding. But I need some advice, because I can't afford to go to the dentist, so I need to know what I can do about this.

My Reply:
Hello,
Thank you for writing in about your problem.

If your gums are already bleeding when you wake up, you better go see your doctor or dentist *immediately. They can give you proper diagnosis and treatment. I can't give you advice, but your physician, periodontist, or dentist can.*

Reader's Reply:
My gingivitis lies mainly at the front set of my teeth. That area of gum is also much darker than the gum at the sides/back which is pink and looks healthy.

I'm just curious as to what changed in the appearance of your gums when they became healthier. Did the color become lighter, pinker, and healthier looking?

I hope that the dentists can stop my gingivitis, I've still yet to go to an appointment, but as long as they can stop it going any further I'll be happy. Each day I look at my gums, I feel they are getting worse and worse, even though I brush my teeth every day. I have actually never tried flossing, because it sounds scary—I can just imagine my gums bleeding from them. BUT I'm prepared to do anything to stop my gums from deteriorating into perodontitis.

Just please tell me there's some hope for my gums to look normal again... even slightly normal! Not pocketed and dark like they are now. What did your gums look like with gingivitis before? And in what ways did they improve? I just want some insight and hope. Thank you!

My Reply:
I totally feel for you. I know how it feels to worry about the health of my teeth and gums. I would hate the idea of losing even one tooth to gum disease. And if several were in danger, I would worry about that much more. My goal is to keep all of my natural teeth for a lifetime.

You have never flossed? That is definitely part of the problem. Daily flossing and brushing are both very necessary to maintain the health of your gums. Learn proper flossing techniques at your dentist's office. Daily removal of the plaque is the key to fighting/preventing gum disease. There are plenty of options that you can discuss with your dentist. [See Chapter 3]

Healthy gums should be a light pink. They should not appear red or puffy at all. There shouldn't be red patches or streaks. And if they bleed and/or have pus, there is definitely a problem.

I think you will find even your dentist will tell you that the outcome of your gum health depends greatly on you and how you care for your gums and teeth at home. The dentist can do some work for you but every person has to be very diligent about gum and tooth care at home.

Your dentist or hygienist will tell you that if you try to rely solely on them to do the work at the office, you will continue to have problems.

It sounds to me like you probably already have periodontal disease. There is hope for your situation. But you need to get professional care right now. Go to a periodontist right away.

❖   ❖   ❖

Gingivitis at Eighteen Years Old

Question:
Eric wrote: Hello, Dave...I have gingivitis and I am only 18 years old...the gingivitis is on my upper row of teeth and it's on 3 of my teeth...everything else is good...but when I brush my teeth, my gums do bleed sometimes...they've bled twice since I switched to a soft bristle tooth brush...my dentist says "u need to floss" which

doesn't do anything...do u think products like Listerine get rid of gingivitis?

My Reply:
Hi Eric. First of all, it is always a good idea to visit your periodontist for diagnosis, treatment, and advice on your gum disease. Age doesn't matter that much with gum disease. Gum health problems have been found in children as young as six years old.

I recently talked to a nineteen-year-old who has a similar problem to yours. He said he did not floss in the past, but he does now. He has already noticed some gum recession. This is a sign of gum disease that is beyond the point of gingivitis. With gingivitis, if you take action, you don't have to lose any gum tissue. Now is your chance to do something before things get worse.

It is my opinion (and experience) that gum disease isn't always resolved by brushing and flossing alone. Having said that, you STILL need to do both. You say flossing does nothing? Actually, it helps to mechanically break up the plaque that is actually responsible for your problems. You need to be flossing—your dentist is right.

Brushing and flossing are both very important for the health of your gums. It is the mechanical breakup of the plaque that is important. You can't just do it once; it has to be done every single day for the rest of your life. Flossing should help you. There are additional tools that you can use as well.

A Perio-Aid and/or a Hydro Floss can be helpful—ask your dentist or periodontist if they are appropriate for you and how to use them. You asked about Listerine? Yes, that can help, too. The ADA (American Dental Association) stands behind Listerine and believes it is proven to prevent the germs that cause gingivitis.

You said, "it's on 3 of my teeth...everything else is good...but when I brush my teeth, my gums do bleed sometimes." It is very seldom that a person has gum disease in only one spot. Usually it is your whole mouth that is affected. You can only see a problem in one spot. However, there is a good chance that there is a lot more going on in your mouth than you are aware of.

You are eighteen, as you mentioned. Now is the time to get busy on this and stop your existing gum disease/gingivitis and prevent it from progressing any further. What you need to do right now is visit a periodontist or dentist—that is your first step. Get a full periodontal evaluation. Thank you for your question, Eric.

※　※　※

Can Sleeping with Your Mouth Open Contribute to Gingivitis?

Question:
I have no gum loss, nor bone loss as per x-rays. I just have really mad gums. However, it is only my four front teeth. The rest of them are fine.

They have been this way for a long time. I live 50 miles from a periodontist. Unfortunately I think I will be getting the UGLY cleaning that I dread! Can they knock you out for it?

I wonder why only my front teeth are affected? My dentist told me I must sleep with my mouth open. Could that cause me to have this problem? I do not think so!

Name Withheld

My Reply:
Yes, sleeping with your mouth open could contribute to the problem.

128

This would create a dry mouth and that is a good time for the bacteria. They can multiply rapidly under such conditions.

Your saliva provides a natural protection as do the mucous membranes of your mouth. When they dry out, it is much easier for the bacteria to reproduce. If you have crowding in the front teeth, that can also contribute to the problem. You definitely want to get rid of these problems.

There is a mouthwash called Biotene, available at most drug stores. It is for combating dry mouth. Check with your periodontist before using it, though. Biotene uses enzymes. When gum disease is more advanced, certain enzymes could actually be harmful. I'm not saying they are the same enzymes that exist in Biotene. I am saying that you need to check with your periodontist before using this mouthwash.

People rarely have gum disease in isolated spots. It is usually a global problem that affects your whole mouth, even though you visibly notice only one area. Go to a periodontist and it is likely that you will find this to be true for you as well.

�֎   �֎   �֎

What about Gum Disease Products for Children?

Question:
Regarding my seven-year-old son: I need to get him to be more consistent at brushing! Do you recommend a child Hydro Floss?

What do you feel is best for a child to use on his/her teeth? I have the same toothpaste you use as well as the mouthwash for gums... How about my other son who is 2?

I am glad, I at least understand that my gums are red and this is NOT normal. I see a lot of people that do not even know they are red, let alone know they have gingivitis, which in the long run can cause health problems. I told my sister. This is so important.

My Reply:
Short answer: Don't use anything for your children's oral health without checking with their dentist first! Xylitol gum might be a good option for your seven-year-old. Xylitol gel might be an option for your two-year-old.

You would apply it to his teeth at bedtime. This gel can often be found at health food stores and it says specifically how to use it on babies. Before I would use any products on my children, I would check with my periodontist or dentist first. If they say it is ok, then by all means—go for it.

You are correct—red, swollen gums are not normal. Just like you, I notice it on people all the time. It is so obvious when you know what to look for. The sad part about it is that they might not even believe you if you told them they had gum disease.

Unfortunately, as many as eighty percent of adults may have it and not even know it. If they did, they would certainly want to do something about it before things really become worse.

Realizing that gum disease exists is the first step. Then, you can think about doing something about it. So many people have some form of gum disease and many don't even know it. It's sad, really.

❖   ❖   ❖

Is There a Deeper Cause to Bleeding Gums?

Question:
I have been experiencing bleeding gums for a few years, and I never paid too much attention to this before.

As yesterday I was having bad breath, I did few things, which worked, and today I am surprisingly better, and I am searching for the answer for what worked and what didn't.

I ate broccoli, nuts, and meat. I did exercises like running, and I cleaned my teeth as usual.

I never read your book, and I am interested if you dig deeper into the problem with gums, because I think that every disease has some spiritual roots and if we use only external things, like pills, it is not the solution.

The real problem is how we live, what we eat, and how we think. Did you find some specific foods or vitamins that help you with gums? I think something is missing in my food, but still cannot find out what.

Thank you. It is good to know that somebody else had the same problem, and solved it already. With all my best wishes to you,
Eva

My Reply:
Hi Eva,
It may shock some of my readers to learn that I actually agree with you that there is a much deeper cause to gum disease and other illnesses. I do believe there is a spiritually related component to health problems. I highly recommend that you read Master Li,

Hongzhi's book, Zhuan Falun. You can download a free copy in the language of your choice at: http://FalunDafa.org

However, I am cognizant that there are two kinds of people in the world: those who believe in spiritual matters and those who firmly believe in the physical world we live in. Unseen and spiritual considerations do not enter into the personal belief systems of the latter. Although, perhaps they should! Not everyone is going to agree with your thoughts on spirituality and disease.

I want to tell you that in physical terms, there is a very good chance that you have gum disease since you have talked about bleeding gums. Of course, you have to go to a dentist to get a diagnosis to confirm that.

In the physical world, the manifestation of anaerobic bacteria is the cause of gum disease of which bleeding gums are but a symptom. Actually, it is the toxins they secrete that cause the problem. Of course, eating the kinds of foods that don't contain processed sugars will mean less food for the bacteria to grow on—they love refined sugar. So, it is definitely better to eat vegetables over sugary snack foods. However, for most people that is not practical and by itself will probably not be enough to stop your gums from bleeding, or get rid of gum disease.

With gum disease, if you already have had bleeding gums for a while, chances are that unless you take some definitive actions, you might find your problems growing. The first thing you really need to do is get evaluated by a periodontist for gum disease. He or she will come up with some treatment recommendations for you. One of those recommendations may very well be to increase your regular professional cleaning schedule to about three months. As individual situations vary, he or she might recommend something a little different. Talk to her about some options for home care [discussed in Chapter 3] *and get approval from your dentist before proceeding with any of them.*

Even dentists and periodontist will admit that the key to your defeating gum disease revolves around what is called home care. Home care includes things like brushing and flossing. But it also can include far more than that.

Perhaps as many as eighty percent of the world's people have some form of gum disease. Many of them brush and floss. I have always contended that brushing and flossing may not always be enough to stop or prevent the worsening of gum disease.

I still hold to that. I use a number of tools to help me combat gum disease. You see, you don't just have to defeat gum disease once and it is over. No. It is a lifetime battle that you must fight EVERY DAY.

As far as food or supplements go—even government websites mention the use of CoEnzyme Q10 in helping to fight against gum disease. Many fruits and vegetables contain vitamin C, which supports healthy gum tissue. Many foods rich in the B vitamins do so as well. Foods such as fish and lean meats may contain zinc, which is considered helpful for healthy gum tissue.

Please remember that it is the daily removal of plaque from your teeth and gum line that is crucial for success in preventing or stopping the progression of gum disease.

I sincerely hope this post was helpful to you, Eva. If not, please feel free to ask a follow-up question.

Warm Regards,
David

※　※　※

Can the Hydro Floss Save My Loose Teeth?

Question:
Hi Dave,

I'm afraid reluctance to visit my dentist regularly has not meant good things. I have gum disease and have used [product name removed] on and off, but have now sensed and sighted tooth movement.

I do not wish to lose my teeth, so I have thought of buying the Hydro Floss—but before I do, please tell me if its use can stabilize or reverse the movement that has started, and the gum receding that is happening.

I am making an appointment with a periodontist now, but would like to have some improvement before I actually go there so as not to bleed too much, and perhaps avoid any surgery.

I am 54 and have excellent teeth but bad gums. The worst is localized top lefthand incisors.

I would appreciate any comments and suggestions.

Rosanne

My Reply:
Hi Rosanne,

I'm afraid that based on the point you are at, you really need to talk to that periodontist. If your teeth are loose, there is a fair chance that he will want to do some gum surgery and add some bone matrix to your damaged area(s). Perhaps Emdogain will be a good option for you.

I do NOT think the Hydro Floss can make a difference for your loose teeth at this point. I do not know how much movement you have, obviously. The Hydro Floss is useful for helping to prevent the buildup of plaque in the first place. However, I do not think you should rely on the Hydro Floss to fix the problem of a loose tooth.

There is a classification of movement that your periodontist will determine. He will take some measurements and check the overall health of your entire mouth's gum tissue. The tissue around every single tooth will be measured for pocket depth and attachment loss. Remember those numbers as they will provide a baseline for you to evaluate your progress in the future.

Do not be afraid to get a little gum surgery. Adding bone to your loose tooth area(s) can firm that tooth up and really help you. I had a gum graft done, as you can read in my book. I tell the story, the surgery was not so bad.

My boss at work had some bone matrix added and it really firmed her teeth up. In other words, the teeth she was having problems with became firm again. She is glad that she had the surgery. She is not going to lose her teeth.

The Hydro Floss can be useful in helping to keep your gums clean and free of plaque buildup to prevent further damage. You will, of course, want to use other tools as well—including your regular dental floss and toothbrush.

The most important thing for you to do now is to visit that periodontist ASAP. You also need to start thinking about how you can improve your home care procedures. You can partner with the periodontist and hygienist to find the best plan for you. Don't buy the Hydro Floss right now. Talk to them about whether it is appropriate for you or not.

Many dentists and periodontists recommend the Hydro Floss to their patients. However, I think your immediate concerns must be addressed first. Go see your periodontist as soon as you can. It's time for you to really get serious in order to keep your teeth for the rest of your life.

After you get things straightened out, I'm sure your doctor will agree that you will need to really be diligent about your home care from now on. At that point, if you aren't told everything they can tell you about home care, ask questions until you have all of your questions answered.

These are your teeth we're talking about, and I know you want to keep them. You'll want to do everything in your power to make sure you do get to keep them. With the right amount of effort at home as well as good professional care on an ongoing basis, I believe you can keep those teeth. You can probably even keep the one that has become loose, too, provided you get it taken care of right away.

Rosanne, I hope this information was useful to you. Please feel free to ask any follow-up questions that you might have.

❊ ❊ ❊

Why has My Tooth Turned Brown?

Question:
This year one of my teeth began to darken. What usually causes that? It has been getting dark even though I brush it. But the teeth next to it are not getting dark. How does just one tooth get targeted like this?

Any suggestions on what you would do if it were you?

Thank you in advance for your reply...

My Reply:
There is a good chance that your tooth has died. However, you will need your dentist to confirm. When an adult's tooth turns brown, it often means the tooth has died. This probably will lead to a root canal and a crown. If a child's tooth turns brown, it is a very different situation.

You should study up a bit on root canals before you get one. There is some interesting information out there. There are some dentists who use special equipment that generates high pressure to insure that all of the canals are sealed properly.

Do you have a question? If you do, please feel free to ask your question here:
                    http://tobeinformed.com/ask-dave-a-question

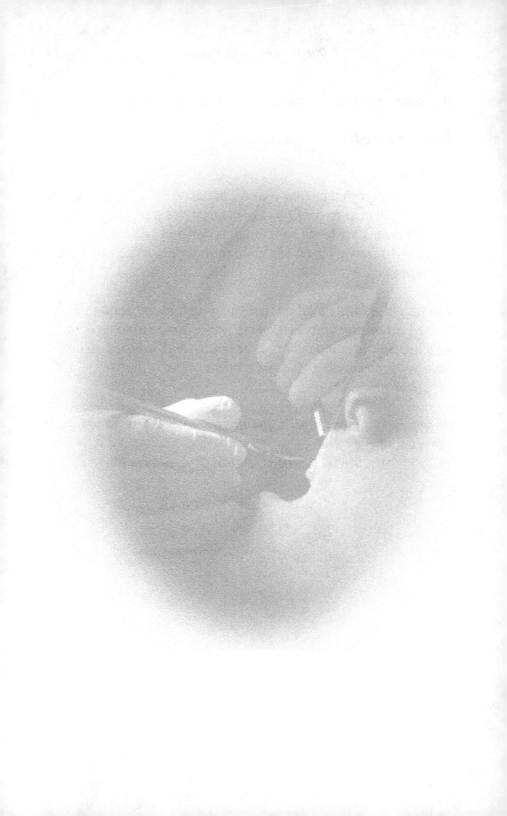

Knowledge,
if it does not determine action,
is dead to us. —Plotinus

The Fight Against
Gum Disease Continues

You Have Been Robbed—Reclaim Your Castle

YOUR SITUATION WITH gum disease did not just appear overnight, and mine did not, either. A long period of ignorance on both our parts has conspired to rob us of healthy gums. Getting your dental health back is not going to happen overnight or because you read this book. There is a final ingredient required: *Action.*

It is easy to think that you just developed gum disease whenever your dental professional informed you about it. Though it could be possible, chances are pretty high that gum disease had been developing in your mouth for a very long time before developing to the stage where it became noticeable. Most people, the vast majority, can stop the progression or prevent it in the first place, provided they do the work.

Recognition of the fact that gum disease did not happen overnight is also crucial to your success. In my case, I can look back and see that my gums bled during dental cleanings for many years. All of that lost time could have been used to stop gum disease from progressing further, preventing it from returning and saving some of my gum tissue. I could have avoided a certain degree of gum recession. I just did not know, and that lack of knowing robbed me. And it either robbed or is still robbing you—or someone you love.

Continual damage slyly built itself up over time. Like a thief in the night, it snuck in the window when you were not looking and hid in your closet. It lurked there for years, slowly tearing holes in the walls and the supporting structure of your home.

Then one day, a building inspector shows up. *Houston, we have a problem brewing here.* The situation is either critical, dire, or just needs some attention on your part. In any case, something has to be done—action has to be taken to make your home's structure sound again and free from further damage.

Fighting gum disease is just like that. You can do the initial work to save your home and evict the robber that was hiding in the closet, and that is all very good and necessary. Once that is accomplished, do not forget to protect your home from undetected entry by another thief. Preventing the return of gum disease is going to require continual effort.

Install alarms—those alarms are your team of professionals. Here is a case in point: I mentioned before that I go in every two months for professional cleanings. During those cleanings, or actually, before they even begin, the hygienist examines my mouth. She tells me if there are any trouble spots. That is my team at work. They let me know if I am missing places while brushing or flossing, and exactly where those places are. Then I know where I need to focus a little extra effort. Sometimes, what they tell me is absolutely amazing—the things I can miss. During this time, I am most interested in finding out if and where any pockets greater than 3 millimeters exist.

Continual Lifetime Action is Needed
to Insure that Gum Disease Does Not Return

Here is an example: One time I went in to get my teeth cleaned, and guess what? I actually had a few pocket depths that were over 3 mm. Do you remember that anything beyond 3 mm is a problem? I had a couple of 4 mm pocket depths.

As hard as I work on my teeth and gums, I still had a problem brewing. I have to admit that I had been slacking a bit, taking short cuts. I was thinking that I had a little wiggle room. You have to stay diligent.

This is one of the great benefits to having a team of professionals working with you. Your hygienist should be your dental health coach. A good hygienist can tell you what you need to pay attention to. She can tell you what you have been missing. Without this coaching, when would I have realized that I had a problem area?

Since I can still have a problem or two, what about you? I added my little story to let you know that preventing the return of gum disease is a lifetime work and requires regular effort on your part. But the alternative is far less attractive to me and I will bet it is to you, too. You and I both want to keep our teeth and smile intact, thank you very much!

You Need a Coach in Your Ring

Let us go a little further with another metaphor. Think of yourself as a professional boxer. You have to fight gum disease. You need a coach. You need people in your corner to support you. But YOU have to go out there and fight. You have to fight daily and you have to win every day. Wow! That is a lot that is being put on your shoulders, isn't it? Now, imagine carrying that burden with no support. No coach. No team. No one to even discuss strategy with. No one watching your back. See the difference? Work smart, not hard. Right?

Sadly, you cannot just stop gum disease once and never have to worry about it again. If we could, that would be a dream come true. If we only had to fight that fight just once, it would be great! Alas, we must enter the ring to the fight against gum disease every day.

Think of this book as part of your support network. Think of it as being there, right inside the comfort of your own home. No dentist is going to come and live with you. No hygienist will either—unless you happen to be married to one. But you have this book. You are not alone, even when at home. Pick it up and read it. You will probably learn something new every time you look at it. This book is one of your team members.

Who else is on your professional team now? Do you have that area of your life handled? The information provided can help you to understand the fight against gum disease a great deal. Your dental professional team however, is more than just a coach. That is your safety net and your primary source of help. Do not go without a coach and support team! You need them.

Professional care is an absolute necessity. You must go to the dentist or periodontist for evaluation, follow up, and to get routine cleanings. Remember the woman who did not know how bad her problem was until she went to the periodontist? By now, you know that I was in the same situation. I just did not know what I was facing.

Furthermore, when I finally did refer myself to a periodontist, I found out that I had a subgingival defect that needed to be fixed. This is something that my dentist seems to have missed. She did not teach me about prevention, either—other than the standard line of "brush and floss."

The standard of care and what insurance will currently pay for is professional cleanings once every six months. Three months is much better for your dental health. You already know that I personally prefer every two months. Work with your dentist or periodontist and his or her recommendations. Sometimes you will find an insurance company that will pay for professional cleanings every three months, but that is a bit rare and could require a special letter from your dentist or periodontist.

Do remember that you have the right to get a second opinion if you do not like what your dentist or periodontist has to say. You can find plenty of other doctors out there. Do not be afraid to walk if you feel uncomfortable or there is an unanswered question mark in your mind. Just like I did when I was told I needed a root canal, and again when my dentist wanted to drill a reversible pulpitis. I am not saying that you should decline a root canal or filling. I am just saying that if you have any doubts—get that second opinion. Once that root canal is complete or the filling installed—you really cannot go back.

Do you think you do not have the time to run around and get a second opinion? Consider that you only get one set of adult teeth. Once you alter them, the change is fairly permanent. Your health is worth the extra effort. Right?

Professionals should be willing to answer all of your questions, patiently and thoroughly, no exceptions. If you are not happy with one professional, go visit another one. Finding someone you trust and are comfortable with is of utmost importance.

When it comes to professional services, we talked in some detail about the drawbacks of placing your trust in a single individual. Finding a good care provider is imperative and worth some effort. You will want to know beyond a shadow of a doubt that your care provider is helping you and looking out for your best interests. It is imperative to find care providers who hold your dental health in high regard and assign great importance to that health.

Work with your dental professional to develop a good home care plan. It is important for you both to be on the same page and for you to have a plan to take care of your teeth and gums at home. Your doctor is your partner in caring for your gums. Work together. A lot can be accomplished that way. Build a winning team! Barring any major traumas, you should be able to keep all of your teeth—if you start in time. With a strong team and your willingness to do the homework that must be done, you can be a continual winner with gum disease.

The War
You probably fully understand by now that there are two major fronts in the war against gum disease. Professional care and home care are the two areas that require battle plans. Just like the United States had to fight in two theaters or two fronts in WWII—Europe and the South Pacific—you also have two fronts in the war. You can pay someone else to fight from the professional side. However, the responsibility for the home care front rests squarely on your shoulders. And you cannot realistically delegate that to anyone else.

In the case of professional care, you can leave that, for the most part, in the hands of your care provider—once you have found a good one that you are satisfied with. Do not skip any regular cleanings, either. They are important for all the reasons previously mentioned and more.

It should be equally clear that professional care alone would not be enough to win the battle against gum disease. You likely recognize by now that you have a personal responsibility to execute successfully, and on a daily basis, a good home care strategy. You probably cannot win the war against gum disease without both of these components firmly in place.

Do Not Fear the Dentist

True, many people fear the dentist, but these are your teeth and gums we are talking about. You have to go—period. Actually, when your gums get healthy again, you will not mind going at all. In fact, you will be excited to get your status checks and to see how well you are doing compared to the past.

I remember the shocked and surprised looks on my dentist and hygienist's faces. I guess they did not expect me to make much progress. That is a moment I will not forget. It was exciting to hear that there was no more bleeding during probing after years of bleeding while getting my teeth cleaned.

They did not quite know what to say. Their faces clearly displayed a look of disbelief. If you can experience a moment like that, then you will know that you have achieved a major accomplishment. You can feel proud at that moment. Take yourself to dinner. You will deserve it. Be sure to remember that the battle against gum disease is life-long and never ends. The only difference is that you will be preventing gum disease, not fighting an active case. Once you get there, things are a lot brighter and a lot easier.

You will have to experiment to see what you can get away with in the way of home care at that point. Everyone is different and no two human beings are facing identical situations. With your two-month or three-month status checks, you will have a gauge to measure your progress, or lack thereof. You will have your fingers on the pulse of your gum disease situation. You will know when something goes wrong and you will know what to do about it.

The game is entirely different at this point. The most dangerous part will be over—now you will just have to maintain. You can do that. If you can defeat it in the first place, preventing the return of gum disease should be easier in comparison. You will have arrived!

However, the battle is still being fought, but the focus is more strongly on prevention now. What a relief that is! Whew, I am glad the worst is over! You will be too.

Actually, I think the worst part is walking around for years not knowing that the damage was accumulating. That was ignorance. In this case, ignorance was not bliss. I wish I knew then what I do now. I hope this book has spared you the abrupt awakening that I had to experience! I also hope you are spared the tissue loss that goes along with letting gum disease exist out of ignorance.

Looking for another good reason to go to the dentist routinely? Remember earlier when I mentioned that the founder of the Mayo Clinic suggested that losing one's teeth would take ten years away from one's life? Wow. Ten years! I want to keep those ten years, don't you?

I know you care about keeping your teeth and conquering gum disease or you would not be reading this right now. I would like for you to keep your teeth, too. We are on the same page—no pun intended. That is the intent of this book, to help you to accomplish the goal of preserving your teeth and gum health. Make sure you have that team of professionals in your corner working to make your fight the best it can be. May you win that battle.

Quick Review of the Basics—Do Not Stop Learning

You have probably heard that repetition is the key to learning. Now it is time to review some of the ground we have traveled. This little review can help you to revisit the key points in your own mind. As you read, you should find yourself naturally gaining greater insight into gum disease.

Do you remember your biology classes in high school or college? Did't have any? Not to worry. This will be easy in comparison. Gum disease is caused by the anaerobic bacteria that grow under the biofilm called plaque. Plaque needs to be removed daily from your teeth and around your gum line. Failure to do this will result in the proliferation of the anaerobic bacteria and gum disease will begin to manifest itself. It is really that simple.

In the beginning, this can manifest as gingivitis. Gingivitis is the fully reversible mild form of gum disease. Your gums can return to a fully healthy state if you take decisive and swift action to remove the problem before it gets any worse.

Not everyone can avoid gum disease; your ability to do so could rely—to a greater or lesser extent—upon genetics and a whole host of other factors. The kind of bacteria that live in your mouth also plays a part in how you are personally affected. Approximately two percent of the population is going to have a difficult time with gum disease, almost regardless of how hard they work to fight or prevent it.

On the other end of the spectrum, two percent of people are virtually immune to developing gum disease. They can do all the wrong things, have terrible home care habits, and still never develop gum disease.

The other ninety-six percent of us can pretty much be successful at fighting, defeating, and preventing the return of gum disease. However, the amount of work required is going to vary from person to person. What that means is that the chances are high that you or someone you love can be successful at stopping the progression of gum disease.

Removing the plaque daily is a lifelong endeavor. The formation of plaque is something that is constantly occurring. When you disrupt the plaque formation, it begins to form again almost right away. Disrupting plaque daily is one of the key concepts in fighting gum disease. Without doing this continually and on a daily basis, your results could be dismal.

The Tools I Have Found to be Useful
In Chapter 3, we visit these tools in detail. This is simply a reminder list.

- The Hydro Floss

- The Mouthwash Cocktail

- Xylitol Gums and Mints

- The Perio-Aid

- AktivOxigen Concentrated Serum—To be used in conjunction with the Hydro Floss. I personally use it by placing eight drops of the serum in the Hydro Floss reservoir prior to using the Hydro Floss.

• Oxygenated Mouthwash—I used this as a substitute for the AktivOxigen Serum or as a regular mouthwash. I believe that its oxygenated compound is powerful for fighting the anaerobic bacteria that cause gum disease. When using it rather than the serum, I would put two capfuls in the Hydro Floss reservoir. Otherwise, I might use it as I would any other mouthwash.

• PerioTherapy Toothpaste

• Essential Oil Compound

• Regular Brushing and Flossing—These cannot be forgotten and must be performed at the rate suggested by your dentist or periodontist.

• Salt Water Rinse

• Scale and Pick Tools -
  Available at your local drug store.

• Sodium or Calcium Ascorbate

• Therabreath or CLÖSYS

• Listerine

• PerioTherapy
  Oral Rinse

*Caution—Do not use any of these products unless your periodontist or dentist has given a nod of approval. Your choice of home care tools should not interfere with your practitioner's plan for your dental health. I am not sure why they would object to any of these tools—but they might. For example, they could possibly not want you to use the Hydro Floss during their initial treatment of your gums. Of course, there could be other scenarios, as well. You need to follow their advice—they are the professionals, after all!

** *The FDA has not evaluated statements or opinions about of any of the products mentioned in this book.*

It Is Up to You from Here on Out!

I hope that you will not just leave things as they are. Study up on gum disease, ask questions. Even the most basic questions will help a care provider understand that you are generally interested in understanding all that you can about protecting your gum health. A genuine and sincere provider should recognize such a spirit in a patient and should do all that he or she can to answer your questions, support you, and help you to understand the big picture. They will respond by telling you more than they will a patient who is just sitting there passively to receive treatment.

Do not be surprised by their surprise over your questions. They are not used to seeing patients who ask for detailed information. Tell them what you already know and let that be a springboard for further discussion and education. Going in with a little bit of knowledge can help them to explain in further detail.

You should feel comfortable enough with your provider to express doubt over his or her treatment plan or the need for any aspect of it. If the care provider acts defensive or indignant, consider finding another one. You do not have time to waste on coddling someone's ego. This is your health we are talking about, and if your care provider can tolerate being second-guessed, patiently accepts and answers your questions, addresses your concerns and replies kindly to your probing—that is a very good sign that you probably have a good practitioner.

Again, your health is arguably one of your most precious assets. You simply cannot afford to blindly trust someone with the health of your gums. You must take responsibility up to the maximum point that you can. These are your teeth, after all. Get a second opinion if your provider leaves you with question marks or if you do not feel comfortable with him or her.

Fighting gum disease is more than just a routine task. In order to be effective, you need to understand everything you can about the problem and the methods that you ultimately choose to combat it with. With such a heart and the backing of your professional team, you can help yourself win the war against gum disease.

Remember that oral and dental disease has been labeled a "silent epidemic." Revisit that phrase in your mind from time to time. Being an epidemic means that it is widespread. The word *silent* reflects the hidden and insidious nature of the disease. Most people do not recognize they have it. Or if they do happen to know, they likely do not understand how badly they have it, or what can happen if they do not take decisive action now!

Left to grow on its own and unchecked, gum disease can overwhelm your defenses and destroy the supporting structure of your gums and teeth. When this happens, gum tissue recedes because there is not enough bone to hold them up. Teeth can become loose when they have little support left.

Right now is the time to start taking action, if you have not already. There is really no time to waste. If you have gum disease, you do not want it to get worse. If you do not have it—which would be outside the norm—then you probably need to take steps to prevent it.

Understand that your gums are like a garden. In order for that garden to bloom and give you the benefit of its best fruits, you have to remove the weeds. The plaque that causes gum disease is the major weed you have to remove. You have to get into that garden daily and remove the weed called dental plaque. Winning the war takes persistent effort. You cannot take a day off, except maybe on rare occasions, or if your care provider tells you to.

One example of a time when your care provider might have you take a break from flossing is if you improperly floss and cut into your gum tissue. There is no reason for this to happen, because flossing should be a gentle event. However, if it does happen at a time when you are just developing your flossing skills, your provider could have you take a day or two off for the benefit of the tissue healing.

Under such a scenario, make sure that you ask the provider if it is okay to use the other tools in your arsenal!

Unfortunately, this war does not end, and you will need to continue fighting it until the day you pass beyond the realm of human life.

Tending your garden and removing the weeds daily is a lifelong endeavor. You cannot just go in to see a dental professional, get your teeth cleaned, and think you are done until your next visit. Diligence in your home care is a must to be successful for both the short and long term.

You cannot ignore your personal responsibilities in this matter without facing the consequences. Even though it is true there is a rare and small percentage of people who generally do not get gum disease—even with the worst oral care habits, and even if they eat the worst possible foods all the time. That is a rare individual and you are probably not in that category.

On the other hand, if you do take care of your gums, both professionally and on your own, you should be able to look forward to a lifetime of healthy gum tissue, as well as getting to keep the teeth that tissue supports. Those who fail to take action could end up without their own natural teeth. Implants or dentures might be the only recourse at that point. I do not relish the idea of taking care of dentures; I have enough to do to get through the day already. Say NO to gum disease and avoid these additional hassles and expenses. Even if you have them, you *still* have to take care of your gums. Having dentures or implants does not spare you that responsibility.

Taking Action is Key

Success at fighting and defeating gum disease requires that a person actually wants to win. The person who does not care, or fails to put in an effort, is not likely to get very far.

Like many things in life, what you put into fighting gum disease is going to be proportionate to the results you get. This will vary from person to person due to a multitude of individual factors. Some people will have to work harder and some will be able to do less. Learning how much work you have to put in is part of your own discovery process, and is to be revealed when you are firmly on the path of fighting gum disease.

With this book, I have attempted to give you the information I think is important to know about gum disease and how to prevent or defeat it in easy-to-understand terminology. I hope that I have succeeded. I have repeated the main concepts in different forms so that by the time you reach the end of the book, you will know what you should about gum disease and what can be done to fight or prevent it.

Basically, the important thing to understand is that home care and professional care are both necessary for the long-term health of your gums. I have told you about the tools I personally use to fight gum disease at home and that I get professional cleanings on an every-two-month frequency. I feel this is extra—but necessary—insurance to make sure that I never have to deal with the consequences of gum disease and the damage it does to my body ever again.

True to what I have mentioned several times, I find that I need to continue with my daily home care to protect the health of my gums. Slacking off does not work. I will notice the health of my gum tissue begin to diminish when I slack off. You should, too.

In my personal situation, since there has been some tissue loss, I need to be sure that no more occurs. I have found that the tools mentioned in this book are very useful to me in maintaining my gum health, just as they were in getting my gums to stop bleeding in the first place.

No Magic Cure
In short, I will repeat that there are no magic bullets. Even the use of chlorhexidine can only be short term. Long term use can cause

trouble. Therefore, there is no way that you can use it all the time. It also requires a prescription to get it in the first place. The staining of your teeth is a side effect of chlorhexidine use. I personally do not want to deal with that, either. You might be different. I think that your care provider will have some objections to you using it all the time anyway.

However, the mouthwash cocktail is fairly powerful and it is made up of common mouthwashes used in series (not mixed together—see the link to directions in Chapter 3). You might find them to be a fairly simple and easy way to improve your dental health, provided your dentist approves the use of these at home.

There are likely to be places along your gum line that you might have a difficult time keeping plaque-free all of the time. This is especially true if you have any crowded or crooked teeth. These are places where stain or plaque will build.

Professional Dental Cleanings

Getting *someone else* to clean your teeth with professional tools can take care of any missed spots or problem areas that are difficult to maintain. This is best done by a professional hygienist who will be working in the office of your periodontist.

You should view your hygienist as a coach—someone who is there to tell you about the spots you are missing. This guidance is very useful. If you do not get it automatically from your hygienist, then ask. The feedback provided could help you develop a better approach to your home care. If everything were really going great, it would be wonderful to know that, as well.

Getting Help with Your Personal Plan

Have an initial meeting with your periodontist and work with him/her to set up a plan that you are confident will work for you. Never be afraid to get a second opinion.

One of the most important aspects of this planning period is that you feel comfortable with the plan so that you will be likely to execute it. Do whatever it takes to insure that you have a workable plan that you feel comfortable with.

A Layman's Guide:
Not a Scientific Work
This is a layman's book and is not intended to exhaustively cover a bunch of science that you would not be interested in anyway. That would be too boring and would not serve you very well. This book is intended to empower you with information about fighting gum disease that you might not be getting from anywhere else.

I hope I have not bored you with my method of delivery. But if I have, please drop me a line and tell me so. You might save readers of future books from the same fate if you just let me know! By the same token, if you feel that you have truly benefited from this information, please let me know.

I tried to use my experiences and those of others to help illustrate key points. While some may find it interesting, I did not write this book for scientists or dental professionals, especially the latter. Those professionals should already know what to do about the health of their own gums. Yet, I would not be surprised if some do not.

I was visiting a local coffee shop and working on this book when a sales professional sitting nearby struck up a conversation with me. He asked what my book was about and, of course, I told him. He described to me how his gums bleed at the dentist's office when they clean them and that sometimes his gums bleed when he brushes or flosses. This is so typical of gum disease. Yet, he did not realize that he had gum disease and, for some reason, his dentist had not told him, either.

This sounds virtually identical to my own story. Rest assured, your gums should not bleed at any time. If they do, that is NOT normal. Check with a periodontist for a diagnosis and recommendations on what to do if that is the case with you. There is a pretty good chance that this guy is suffering from some form of gum disease. He does not know it, and no one told him—except me. Of course, he needs a professional diagnosis to confirm that there really is gum disease there. Why do you think it is that no one has informed him that he has a problem?

For most people in a similar situation as our friend above, gum disease should not be that hard to deal with. The problem is that, left unchecked, problems will grow in size and scope over time. Then one day, they will give it a label.

At that point, you might feel that this just sprung up overnight. The fact is, it probably did not just suddenly appear. It has been there for years and only now are the symptoms getting bad enough that they feel something has to be done—then they label it. Why not do something now and avoid getting to that stage in the first place?

If I had started earlier, I could have avoided some gum recession. A lack of recession adds to an attractive smile and a more youthful appearance. Severely receded gums are not attractive.

You may have noticed this in others already.

Read it Again

You have most likely heard form other sources besides me that repetition is the key to learning. With that in mind, do not just leave things here. Go back and read this book again. Read it as many times as you can.

You are bound to pick up new information each time. Ultimately, with repeated study, you will begin to understand the 'big picture' of gum disease and both the why and the how will become crystal clear at some point. Again, remember that repetition is the key to learning.

If you are a bit foggy on everything right now, do not worry; that is normal. Keep going, keep learning, keep reading, and do not be afraid to consult other sources, as well. Do everything you can to enhance your knowledge of gum disease. This will help keep you motivated to keep on fighting or preventing gum disease for the long term.

You only get one set of permanent teeth as far as we know. There is really no substitute for having your own natural teeth. They are best suited to do the job they were created for. You might remember my story of the older man at a New Year's Eve party who said, "of course my gums are receding, I'm getting old."

You might realize at this point that I do not agree with that statement at all. His gum recession is most likely due to gum disease or possibly brushing too hard.

A popular clinic's website suggests that ninety-five percent of people have gum disease by the age of sixty-five. You have to work very hard to prevent it, and if you already have it you will want to work hard to stop its progression. Then, you will want to work hard to prevent that progression from starting again. Keep this book. It is a lifelong companion for fighting gum disease.

Now—It Is Your Turn!

Basically, the bottom line is that the rest is up to you from here on out when it comes to fighting or preventing gum disease. Knowledge is power, but knowledge without action is merely potential power. If that potential never translates to reality through action, it is practically useless to you.

You can read my latest posts and thoughts on gum disease at my blog:

http://tobeinformed.com/category/gum-disease/

I tried to cover as much as I possibly could with a little repetition built in. However, if something still is not crystal clear, you can ask me questions. At my blog there is a link that says, "Ask Dave a Question." It will take you to this page:

http://tobeinformed.com/ask-dave-a-question

If your question is selected, it will be answered and posted on the ToBeInformed.com website under the category mentioned above. If you leave your email address, I will even write to you and let you know the exact link to your question and its answer

Do you think others could benefit from this book? I certainly hope you do. If you have found this book useful, share it with others. Tell them the information you now have. Explaining it to someone else will not only help them learn, but will help you as well! When you try to explain this to someone else, you will inevitably learn more yourself.

Remember that as many as eighty percent of adults are walking around this planet with some form of gum disease right now—that is commonly agreed upon by professionals. This is a virtual tragedy that does not need to be. Spread the word. Help others. It will just make our world that much better.

I really hope this book served you by taking some of the mystery out of gum disease. You tell me—has it? I am pretty sure it has. I also hope you feel empowered at this point. Remember that the two main aspects to succeeding against gum disease are professional care and home care. You really need both. One without the other just is not going to work. The last ingredient you need is personal determination. Steel your will to do what it takes to bring your gums back to a healthy state!

*A happy life
consists in tranquility of mind.* —Cicero

The Mind-Body Connection

A BOOK ABOUT a health related subject cannot be considered complete without a section that discusses the relationship between the mind (your thoughts) and the body (your home). There is a tough leap that has to occur in a person's mind to connect something that manifests in concrete ways, like gum disease or cancer, to the state of one's mind. I am certainly not advocating that positive thinking will always conquer disease. Yet, it has been interesting to note that the subjective experiences of many people seem to indicate that the mind does have influence over the health of our bodies.

I offer you the story of Bernie Siegel—a surgeon who discovered some truths about healing that you probably will not find in many medical school texts or curriculums. Stories similar to Bernie's are out there. They do not enter the mainstream media or educational channels as often as they occur, for some reason. However, they do exist, and whether mainstream society tries to ignore these stories or not has no bearing on the truth that exists within them.

I wrote the following article a couple of years ago. You can find it at various places on the Internet. It has also appeared in the *Epoch Times Newspaper*: http://en.epochtimes.com.

How to Benefit from the Mind-Body Connection

Dr. Bernie Siegel, author of *Love, Medicine and Miracles*, was once a distraught surgeon who fretted over his inability to effectively serve his cancer patients. Dr. Siegel's recognition and growing understanding of the mind-body connection eventually allowed him to serve his patients and himself in a greater capacity.

Bernie writes in his book, "When a doctor reports amazing improvements in a patient's condition, he or she almost never mentions that person's beliefs and lifestyle, but when I inquire, I find the patient always has made some drastic change toward a more loving and accepting outlook. The patient seldom tells an unreceptive doctor about this, however."

When the person's mind changed, the state of their health changed. Hence, the importance of the mind-body connection.

However, just covering up the surface with positive thinking isn't necessarily going to help. It is like cleaning out a house. The dirt and filth have to be removed and the stale air replaced with fresh air. There has to be a fundamental change for real healing to take place. Surface level positive thinking is not going to affect this kind of change, just like lightly dusting our homes will not get the real dirt out.

So, what are the dirty and stale things in our minds? Well, they could be things like grudges, prejudices, anger, resentment, and hate. One spiritual principle from religion talks about "loving your enemy." That can't be done without giving up hate. By giving up something bad, we can make room for something good to come in and may, as a result, see a corresponding change in our bodies.

The problem here is that many of these bad things are buried and hidden and we will not necessarily see them or recognize them in ourselves. We can be certain that they are there, though; it is a virtually inevitable consequence of living in a world that is more focused on selfishness and less concerned with loving others.

So, finding these bad things and eliminating them requires intro-spection; it requires looking at oneself hard and long. However, there is still a problem. When we are searching within our minds, we have to have a standard to do the comparison with. Otherwise, how will we find anything? How will it stand out?

Let's look to one of the greatest thinkers of the Western world, Socrates. What did Socrates do with his life? Didn't he teach others about virtue? Socrates talked about things like absolute goodness, beauty, and truth. Interesting, isn't it? One of the most influential people in western thinking emphasized virtue to his students.

If someone as great, as well loved and respected as Socrates thought these things were important, perhaps therein lies the key to the mind-body connection. To live a truly healthy and worthwhile life, maybe virtuous thoughts like truth and goodness are what our minds should embrace, rather than the negative things modern life finds us clinging to.

Remember what Bernie said: "I find the patient always has made some drastic change toward a more loving and accepting out-look." When we embrace truth and goodness, the beauty of life and this vast universe that we live in becomes evident. Perhaps that is when we can heal our bodies. Healing can happen and flow from the mind.

This article is for information purposes only. It is not meant to diagnose, prevent, or treat any illness or health issue. If you have or think you might have a health condition, please visit your primary-care physician immediately for diagnosis and treatment.

You Go Where Your Head Goes

My father used to teach us that "you always go where your head goes." He meant that purely in the physical sense as he taught us boys a little too much about rough-housing indoors, to the dismay of my mother—whose main concern was to protect the peace, and her household, from damage.

Yet, there are ever greater dimensions to Dad's favorite saying. Your mind and body come and go together. Therefore, your thoughts, notions, emotions and yes, attitudes, affect your body and can also affect your body's health.

Attitude

You might have read Charles Swindoll's near-famous work titled, "Attitude." Perform an Internet search for "Charles Swindoll Attitude," and you will quickly find his little masterpiece. You often see plaques with his quote in cubicle walls throughout corporate America, and elsewhere.

The all-important point about attitude is that it is the one thing you have a very large degree of control over. You have very little control over many aspects of life. You cannot determine when it is your time to pass beyond this realm. You cannot always control the good or bad fortune that visits you. You cannot often stop unforeseen tragedies. You probably cannot wake up as the President of the United States tomorrow morning just by wishing for it.

Despite all of the popular self-help talk being bandied about suggesting that you have ultimate control over your reality—the fact is, you really do not have that much control over external factors. Not so for your attitude. You can exert a great deal of control over how you view what happens to you. Attitude is a powerful tool to improve or, conversely, to harm ourselves with. This gives the term "self-destruction" a whole new twist, doesn't it?

Attitude is contagious. When you have a good one, you can share it and people will love you for it. You can probably remember a time when you felt very euphoric; your positive energy was overflowing and everyone you talked to responded favorably to you. You have probably also experienced the opposite, a time when you were not in a good mood, perhaps a bit down and maybe even irritable. People do not smile as much towards you when that kind of mood presides over you, do they?

Upon reflecting carefully on this, you could come to the conclusion that if this really is the sole thing we have control over, it must be of utmost importance. Free will is something we all have. Bernie has shown us that your mind, your outlook, and your attitude can influence a serious disease like cancer. Isn't that amazing? What other areas of your life might benefit from an examination and overhaul of your thoughts, notions, and emotions?

Falun Dafa Exercise & Teachings Improve Both the Mind and Body
The practice, teachings, and exercises of Falun Dafa, also known as Falun Gong, are truly extraordinary! FalunDafa.org is a large

website with lots of resources. Go there and learn as much as you can about it.

In particular, the book, *Zhuan Falun*, has helped me to heal deep hurts that reside within my mind and heart. In addition, it has helped me to focus on truthfulness, compassion, and tolerance—three things our world could definitely use a lot more of, right?

Some of the subjective health benefits and experiences of Falun Gong practitioners has been documented in a book called, *Falun Gong Stories: the Journey to Ultimate Health.* You can read the entire book, edited by two medical doctors, online at the following address:
http://clearwisdom.net/emh/download/publications/
health_index.html

You will find free video instructions of the Falun Gong exercises in English at this web address:
http://www.FalunDafa.org/eng/exercises.htm

Since the focus of the practice is on truth, compassion, and tolerance, it can automatically fill your mind with positive, good things. Remember the lesson learned from Bernie's experience and what Socrates' teachings consisted of? Focus on the good and positive and see what happens next!

Unfortunately, this beautiful, life affirming practice called Falun Gong is being brutally persecuted in China at the time of this writing. You can read more about the persecution at:
http://faluninfo.net

You might also wish to do your part to help stop the persecution. Learn more about what you can do at: http://fofg.org

Our minds are like a garden. To have a beautiful and wonderful garden filled with the things you love and enjoy, you will want to keep the weeds out. Embrace the beautiful things. A life affirming practice like Falun Dafa can supercharge your garden!

Life is Incredibly Short

For those of you who get a chance to read this, know one thing: Life is short. It will be over in the blink of an eye and when it is, so many things just will not matter.

What will matter? Any kindness towards others that you show now will be remembered forever. There is an infinite payoff to being nice, and you should definitely do it.

It is easy for our own troubles and problems to get us down. It is a tough world out there—no doubt about it.

Be good to others is the best advice there is. And if you can be tolerant toward others—even when they have wronged you—you are a superior person. This tolerance cannot be surface level. It has to come from the heart. Read Zhuan Falun. It is the best book I know of.

Warm Regards,
Dave Snape

P. S. Your feedback on this book would be most welcome. You can give your feedback at the same page where you can ask questions: http://tobeinformed.com/ask-dave-a-question. Please let me know if I may have your permission to post your comments to my websites.

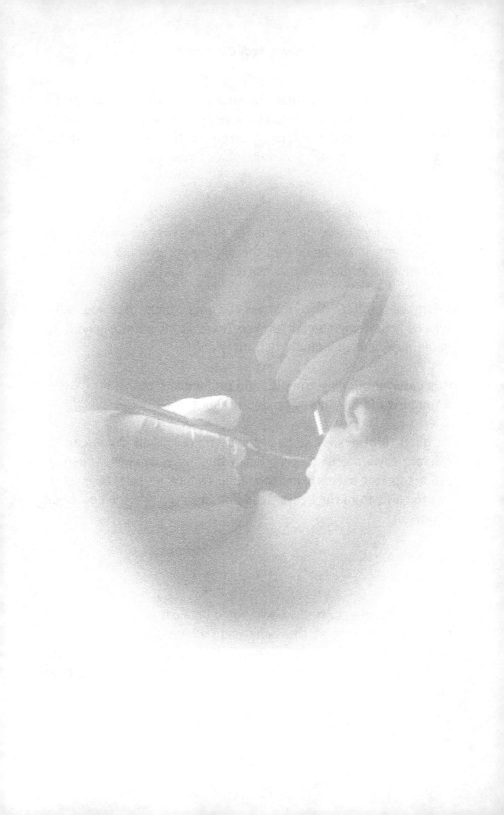

References

Can eating hard cheese strengthen your tooth enamel? The answer is yes based on a November 1991 study published in the Journal of Oral Rehabilitation (PMID 1762023). The Dental Research Unit of Hadassah Medical School located in Jerusalem, Israel conducted this study—Eating hard cheese may harden tooth enamel. In this study, cola was used to weaken the enamel. Hard cheese was eaten by the subject participants and their teeth where examined again. The effect was verified via scanning electron microscopy (SEM), which is basically a way to observe far smaller things than optical microscopes are currently capable of.

The Effect of Oral Irrigation with a Magnetic Water Treatment Device on Plaque and Calculus (ISSN 0303-6979)—Study on the effectiveness of the Hydro Floss found in the May 1993 issue of the *Journal of Clinical Periodontology.*

Up To 80% of Adult Americans Have Some Form of Gum Disease: U.S. Public Health Service, National Center for Health Statistics. Periodontal disease in adults, United States 1960-1962. Washington, DC: Government Printing Office; 1965. PHS publication number 1000, Series 11 No. 12—A study on working adults showed that 85% of men ages 18-64 had some form of gingivitis and 79% of women. Subsequent surveys have shown lower numbers.

National Institute of Health Website Cites the 80% gum disease figure: At the time of this writing it said, "About 80 percent of U.S. adults currently have some form of the disease. It ranges from simple gum inflammation, called gingivitis, to serious disease that results in damage to the bone."

http://www.nlm.nih.gov/medlineplus/gumdisease.html

Here is another reference on a NIH site about the 80% figure: "If you have been told you have periodontal (gum) disease, you are not alone. An estimated 80 percent of American adults currently have some form of the disease.

Periodontal diseases range from simple gum inflammation to serious disease that results in major damage to the soft tissue and bone that support the teeth. In the worst cases, teeth are lost.

Gum disease is a threat to your oral health. Research is also pointing to possible health effects of periodontal diseases that go well beyond your mouth (more about this later). Whether it is stopped, slowed, or gets worse depends a great deal on how well you care for your teeth and gums every day, from this point forward."

Location at the time of this writing:
http://www.nidcr.nih.gov/OralHealth/Topics/GumDiseases/
PeriodontalGumDisease.htm

The Mayo Clinic website suggests that **95% of people over 65** may have some form of Periodontal (gum) Disease. Location at the time of this writing:
http://www.mayoclinic.org/news2006-rst/3333.html

If nothing else, this reinforces that gum disease is serious and you have to really work to prevent it.

Mayo Clinic— "...nearly 80 percent of American adults have some form of gum (periodontal) disease." Location at the time of this writing: http://www.mayoclinic.com/health/gingivitis/DS003631

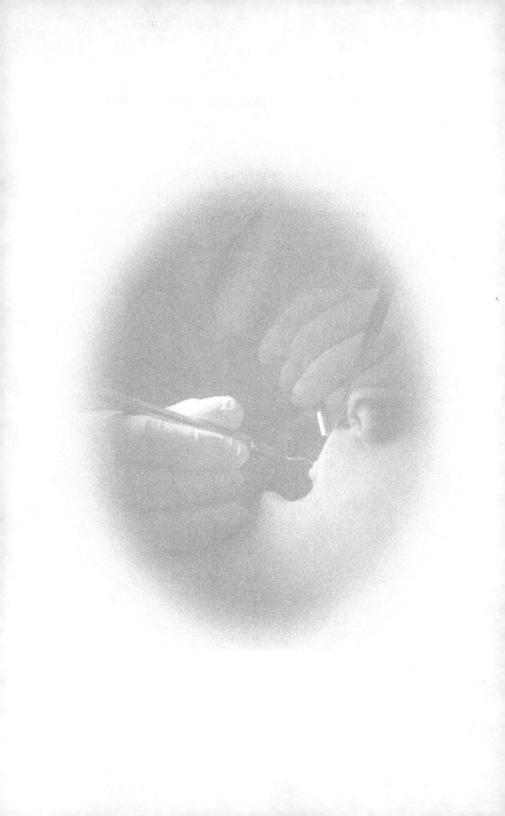

Gum Disease Resources

American Academy of Periodontology website—This is a gem of a website for gum disease information. It can help you find a periodontist as well. The web address is: http://www.perio.org/ It even has a gum disease self-assessment survey. However, you really must see a periodontist in person.

NIH—National Institute of Health Website on Gingivitis: http://www.nlm.nih.gov/medlineplus/ency/article/001056.htm

A Report on Techniques for Regrowing Bone for the Purpose of Placing Dental Implants. This is heavy reading with pictures and strong support for the notion of keeping your teeth in the first place: http://www.perio.org/resources-products/pdf/lr-bone-augmentation.pdf

Epidemiology of Periodontal Diseases—You will be surprised to learn that many school age children already have gingivitis–the amount has ranged from 40% to 60% in different national surveys.

Location: http://www.perio.org/resources-products/pdf/48-epidemiology.pdf

Tools

Xylitol Gums and Mints: http://tobeinformed.com/xylitolgum

The Hydro Floss Oral Irrigator: http://tobeinformed.com/421/

AktivOxigen Concentrated Serum:
http://tobeinformed.com/oxygen-serum

PerioTherapy Formulas for gum health:
http://tobeinformed.com/perio-formula

PerioTherapy Oral Rinse: http://tobeinformed.com/perio-rinse

PerioTherapy Toothpaste: http://tobeinformed.com/perio-tooth-paste

PerioTherapy Gum Care System:
http://tobeinformed.com/gum-care

Essential Oil Blend (available Internationally):
http://tobeinformed.com/oils

Alternative Gum Disease Model—There are voices that run contrary to mainstream opinions on virtually every topic, and the topic of gum disease is no exception. I have read Dr. Gerard Judd's book, and can only tell you that it presents a very different model for dental care—it is very far from mainstream views. I will offer no comment on the information presented or its validity, with one exception: I tried the sodium ascorbate rinse he discusses in his book and it appears to have had a good effect on my gum tissue. If you decide to read his book, proceed with caution and do not do anything without consulting your dentist first. The name of Dr. Judd's book is *Good Teeth, Birth to Death*.

Other Health Resources

Falun Dafa—http://FalunDafa.org. I believe this to be the foundation of my personal health regimen. You can read about people who have subjectively experienced what they believe to be profound healing experiences from this powerful qigong practice from China.

Two MDs have edited a collection of such stories. The book was edited by William Franklin McCoy, MD, and Lijuan Zhang, MD, PhD and published by Golden Lotus Press.

The name of the book is: *Falun Gong Stories: A Journey to Ultimate Health.*

You can read *A Journey to Ultimate Health* online for free here: http://clearwisdom.net/emh/download/publications/ health_index.html

Nasal/Sinus Irrigator—Created by an Ear, Nose, and Throat (ENT) medical doctor, many believe the Hydro Pulse has helped them with their chronic nasal and sinus issues. The Hydro Pulse may also be useful for those who work in construction or for those who breathe dust or fine particulate matter as a consequence of their occupation. I read that Patient Care Magazine stated that using the Hydro Pulse in some cases caused some patients to no longer need medication for their chronic sinusitis. The Hydro Pulse is a device that is registered with the USFDA and insurance will often accept billing for it. The insurance billing code for the Hydro Pulse is K0183.

You can find a Hydro Pulse or similar device here: http://tobeinformed.com/hydropulse

The Book: *Natural Cancer Treatments that Work*—I have this book and the extras that go with it. You can find it at http://tobeinformed.com/natural. There are a lot of stories in the material that comes with this book of people who have either stopped or caused their cancers to go into remission using natural means. The main book is over 400 pages of reference material. There is an incredible amount of information in this book!

Here is an interesting fact. Most of the medicines that we have today are synthetic concentrated copies of what already exists in Mother Nature. They add a few twists to make it into something they can patent. Or, they patent the synthetic process. Anyway, these things are mostly derived from naturally existing plant chemicals which are also know as phytochemicals. This is a something that many people are not aware of.

Of course, with something as serious as cancer, it is advised that you work closely with your physician. Do not make a move without consulting with your physician on this serious disease or any other illness. If you have a progressive doctor, he may allow you to try some of these. Never forego proper medical treatment from a licensed doctor. If it is true for gum disease, then it is doubly or even triply true for something as serious as cancer. This is your LIFE we are talking about. So please, please, do not think that book, this book, or any other book is a substitute for professional medical care. One major reason is that the natural things could interfere with or have violent reactions with the things that your doctor is using to treat you. It is super-important that you work with a physician on something as serious as cancer. I would not want you to rely solely on anything independent of qualified professional advice. At the same time, do not close your mind off to the idea of natural alternatives.

National Institutes of Health Website: http://www.nih.gov/— Health Topics from A-Z.This is a US government institution. It is a good place to view what is acceptable from a mainstream medical point of view. You can often find some information on medicinal properties of plants and herbs as well.

The Water Cure Website: http://www.WaterCure.com—This site was created based on the work of an MD. His opinion is that water is far more important than most realize. He has seen drinking a few glasses of water work miracles. He first noticed this effect in an Iranian prison. A prisoner bent over in pain seemed to be very ill. After this doctor gave him several glasses of water, his symptoms went away.

When I was a student, I clearly remember my biochemistry teacher giving his opinion on what people should do to optimize their health. He stated that everyone should drink a gallon of water per day and take some brewer's yeast every day.

I have noticed that I have much more energy and generally feel better when my state of hydration increases—when I am drinking more water. Hydration can have an effect on virtually everything from physical strength to your mood.

Maybe you have tried drinking more water before. Starting and maintaining an increased intake of water is difficult, isn't it? I have found a little trick that might help. I drink water after I swish it around my mouth first, allowing it to mix with my saliva. You could be surprised by what a difference this makes. You may suddenly discover that you really are thirsty, and will naturally want to drink more water.

I think that when we drink water without mixing it with saliva for a few moments, it is uncomfortable to drink and you may not even believe you are thirsty. Once I started using this method, I was able to drink far more water than ever before. I discovered that I really was thirsty for water. Things changed. My body seemed to work better. I felt more energy. A very mild coating on my tongue started to dissipate. My teeth seemed cleaner. Of course, this is all subjective; I acknowledge that.

I've read before that you are physically stronger when you are fully hydrated. I believe that is true. Actually, it seems to me that a whole host of body processes should work better when you have an adequate (or better) intake of water. Feeling down? Feeling blue? Feeling a lack of energy? Maybe more water will create a shift in those states.

Be sure to check with your health care provider before modifying your intake of food or water, or before changing your level of exercise.

Vision Improvement: I have dabbled with vision improvement therapies at various times throughout my life. At one time, I had a prescription that was −3.5 diopters in one eye and −3.25 in the other eye. Last time I went in, my vision needed −2.5 diopters in each eye to correct to 20/20 vision. I convinced the doctor to bump me down to −2.25 in each eye to decrease near point strain and to give some room for improvement. Does natural vision improvement work? It is really hard to say, but my prescription has decreased somewhat over the years. That was some very sporadic dabbling in vision improvement. What I have always lacked is a structured program. Now, I have found one and am currently giving it a try to see what happens. At the time of writing this, I am on day four of the program. I have committed to writing about it on my blog for at least twenty-five consecutive days. If you want to read about my journey, visit: http://tobeinformed.com/vjourney. Who knows, maybe I will have some good news to report by the time you get this.

Home Foot Spa Detoxification—KellyAnn Andrews has told me an amazing story about a woman who had terrible lead toxicity. She was an artist who worked with stained glass. After her first footbath, they had the water analyzed and found thirty units of lead in it. If you would like to read more about KellyAnn and her scientifically proven foot spa devices, visit: http://tobeinformed.com/footbath

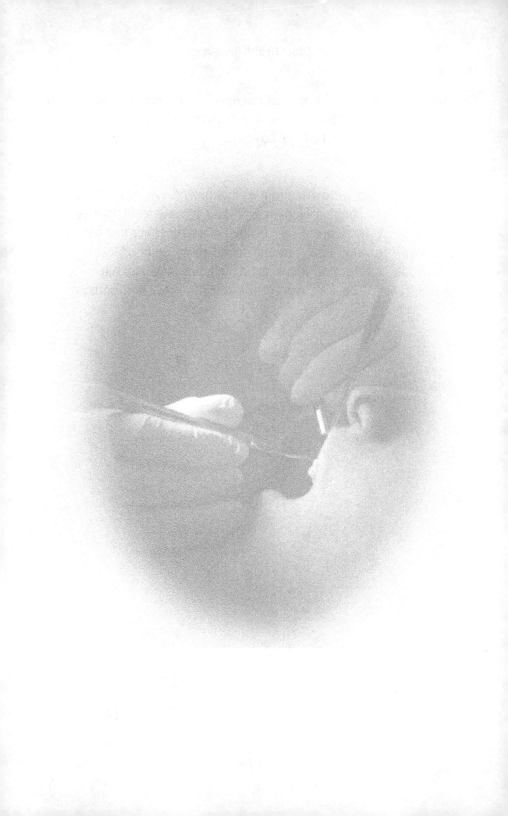

Final Notes

As far as gum disease goes, I hope this book went a very long way to empowering you with knowledge and understanding that you did not previously have.

What You Should Know about Gum Disease should not be reproduced by anyone or by any means without the specific written permission of the author.

However, copies of the articles in the appendix only may be reproduced electronically or in print so long as the author's byline that appears at the end of each article is included with that article wherever it is used. Electronic publications should include active hyperlinks in the author's byline. You may send copies of the articles to friends under the same conditions.

As a reminder: nothing in this book should be construed as advice. Though I have made every attempt to make sure the information is correct and accurate, I cannot guarantee that it is. That is especially true when you consider that even experts have differing viewpoints. Current information might also change in the future.

This book was not intended to provide advice about gum disease or any other health condition. This book is for information and entertainment purposes only. You should seek diagnosis, treatment, advice, and care from a periodontist or other dental professional if you have or think you might have gum disease or any other oral health problem. For non-oral health problems, visit a physician for advice, diagnosis, and treatment. The United States FDA has not evaluated statements about any of the products mentioned in this book, nor have they evaluated the opinions of the author. You are further cautioned not to utilize the information in this book for any practical purpose unless specifically told to do so by a physician, periodontist, or dentist, and then, solely as a result of their instructions to you and not as a result of it having been written about in this book.

Appendix:
Articles for Reprint

If I have done any deed worthy of remembrance,
that deed will be my monument.
If not, no monument
can preserve my memory. —Agesilaus the Second

> **Note:** This appendix is for those who want to help others find out more about gum disease and the information in this book. There is no new information here and the articles are redundant in nature. They are simply included for those who might wish to publish them on their blogs, websites, and magazines. If you want to strengthen your knowledge and understanding about gum disease further, these articles may not be helpful. Instead reread Chapters 1 through 6 to gain greater understanding.

Think of all the people in the world who are suffering right now with gum disease and do not have a clue on what to do about it. Some are not even aware that they have it. If we can catch them before things get too bad, maybe they can be spared the agony and consequences of gum disease that has run rampant in others for far too long. Wouldn't it be great to help even one person avoid massive gum recession and/or tooth loss? Wouldn't it be wonderful to empower them to save their hard-earned money from being spent on costly treatments over something that could have been avoided? Wouldn't it be great to prevent someone from having to get expensive implants or dentures?

If you are a person who sees value in helping others, then this will make total sense to you. If you are the kind of person who understands this, if you see the BIG picture, then know that this appendix was designed to help you spread the word.

What you will find here is a collection of articles I have written to help others find out about gum disease. These articles could seem a bit redundant to you. They are. Although, if you have had trouble grasping the information you have read so far in this book, or would just like a refresher, then it might be a good idea to read a couple of these articles to help reinforce key concepts.

For most people, the progression of gum disease can be stopped, and gum disease can also be prevented in the first place. People should know this. It should not be a hidden mystery. Lack of understanding these simple concepts can bring misery to people.

If you are still with me at this point, let me explain what you can do to help. What you will find in this appendix is a series of articles. You have my permission to print them on your website, blog, bulletin board, magazine, book, etc. You can even print them out and share them with friends and family. You can fax them, mail them, submit them to magazines, whatever you think is appropriate. Please use good taste when doing so. The only other requirement is: wherever you use one of these articles, you must include the author byline found at the end of each article.

To clarify what the author byline is, I have included an example here:
David Snape is the author of the book, *What You Should Know about Gum Disease*. You can find Dave and ask questions about gum disease or other health, fitness, or wellness topics at:
http://whatyoushouldknowaboutgumdisease.com

That is the requirement. You have permission to print the articles in this appendix (and only from this appendix) pretty much anywhere so long as you follow the guidelines and use good taste in where you display them. You can find these articles and the tool at:

http://tobeinformed.com/gdarticles

Here are the articles, arranged in no particular order:

Gingivitis is Serious

Gingivitis and what it can evolve into are responsible for the majority of tooth loss in the world. Most of us would very much like to avoid the use of false teeth or implants. At a New Year's Eve party, one man said to us, "There is no substitute for your own teeth."

Gingivitis is silent; it sneaks up on us. It can be virtually invisible, causing little or no trouble for years. Then one day, we realize that our gums have receded to the point where something has to be done or we will lose a tooth or teeth.

We then must go to a periodontist and spend large amounts of cash to make things right again, if possible. The bone and supporting tissue structure can often be restored, but it takes some work and expense to make that happen. The results might not be ideal. A lot of people, both professional and nonprofessional, believe the damage that can be caused by gingivitis is often preventable.

Do you believe that brushing and flossing are enough to prevent gum disease? Why do so many people with seemingly good oral care habits still get gingivitis? In fact, a large proportion of people all over the world are suffering from some degree of gingivitis or periodontal disease right now.

Even if we just focus on the countries that have abundant supplies of readily accessible dental floss and toothpaste, it still holds true that too many suffer from some form of gum disease.

Approximately two percent of people are not going to get gingivitis; they seem to have a natural immunity to it. That leaves ninety-eight percent of us who could experience some form of gum disease, either mild or severe, in our lifetimes.

The vast majority of tooth loss is due to gum disease. So how do we take better care of our gums?

Part of the answer could be in oral irrigation. Shooting a stream of water around the neck of the tooth might help to clean the gum tissue, removing harmful bacteria and reducing plaque build up.

When the bacteria form colonies around or below the gum line, it can irritate the gums, causing them to pull away from the tooth. When this happens, the entire structure, including the bone that supports the tooth, will begin to erode.

As time goes by, the gum tissue can pull further away from the tooth, creating even greater opportunities for bacteria to exploit. See how this might become a vicious cycle? The problem can feed upon itself.

However, many people believe that a daily cleaning around the neck of the tooth with a jet stream of water will help to control gum disease. If this were true, wouldn't it be worth it to use an irrigator?

To give you an example of how severe this problem can become, a woman recently wrote to me and told me that she finds blood in her mouth when she wakes up in the morning because her gums bleed. If anyone is in a situation like this, she should go to a dentist or doctor immediately. This is a serious situation and needs to be addressed professionally, as soon as possible.

Actually, if you have or believe you might have gingivitis, or any other health condition, you should consult your dentist or doctor for diagnosis and treatment right away.

David Snape is the author of the book, *What You Should Know about Gum Disease*. You can find Dave and ask him questions about gum disease or other health, fitness, or wellness topics at:
http://whatyoushouldknowaboutgumdisease.com

Gum Disease and Dental Checkups
About a year ago, my dentist and hygienist said that I had gum disease. Actually, I suspect that I have had it for over a decade. The interesting thing about gingivitis is that it does not make much noise as it slowly erodes your gum tissue. Sometimes, a lot of bone loss can occur before you become aware of it.

What made me pay attention was when a hygienist wanted me to sign a paper that the office would not be responsible if I lost my teeth. At first, I saw this as a possible marketing ploy, since they wanted me to have a root scaling and planing procedure done. That sounded painful and expensive.

I figured that having me sign that paper was part of their attempt to move me in the direction of accepting this treatment. They wanted me to start right away. I declined. I was not about to approve a treatment that sounded so serious without a little investigation of my own.

What I found was disturbing. I think that a lot of people do not quite understand that bleeding gums, no matter how minute the bleeding, is a bad sign. For example, I have heard someone say that their gums only bleed if they push too hard with a toothbrush. She thinks that means she does not have gingivitis or gum disease.

However, you would have to push fairly hard to make healthy gum tissue bleed. Therefore, if a person has gums that bleed from brushing or flossing, there is a chance that person has gum disease. A person who notices bleeding gums should check with a dentist for diagnosis and treatment.

I also discovered that a scaling and root planing was not something I wanted, either. In fact, a relative of mine had the procedure done. In her opinion, it made her gums worse. The procedure involves numbing the gum tissue and scraping underneath the gum line and down the root to remove any built-up tartar or plaque.

I researched some possible alternative solutions and found something I thought might be promising. I tried it, and by the next visit my gums had become healthier. They were better to the point that the hygienist and dentist said that there was no more tartar under the gum line. I no longer needed that root scaling and planing treatment.

I recently visited the dentist again and they said my gums are continuing to improve. This time there was zero bleeding during the probing part where they check for pocket depth with a metal instrument. No bleeding during a checkup is a good sign.

Gingivitis can be hazardous to your health. Infected gums can provide a pathway for bacteria to enter the blood stream. In addition, gum disease is the major cause of tooth loss, not cavities, as one might expect.

If you have or think you might have gingivitis, gum disease, or any other health problem, be sure to visit your doctor or dentist for proper diagnosis and treatment.

David Snape is the author of the book, *What You Should Know about Gum Disease.* You can find Dave and ask him questions about gum disease or other health, fitness, or wellness topics at:

http://whatyoushouldknowaboutgumdisease.com

Gingivitis is a Funny Topic

"Gingivitis is a funny topic." That is what my friend at work told me when I mentioned my website. "I don't think so," I thought. Gingivitis and gum disease are serious. They can cause a person to lose his teeth. Many, many people have gingivitis and/or gum disease. A lot of those people do not even know it.

A person often finds out he has gum disease after a lot of gum tissue has receded and has been lost. Unfortunately, it is expensive and difficult to restore the gum tissue when it gets to that point. But why let things get that bad in the first place? It is not difficult to defeat gingivitis. It is even easier to prevent it.

So why haven't you heard how to do it, then? That it is a difficult question to answer. On the one hand, people usually do not even recognize that they have gingivitis in the first place. On the other hand, many dental professionals are very busy seeing patients. Perhaps teaching prevention is low on their priority list. They spend their time putting out the fires that arise from the consequences of gum disease instead. Unfortunately, if you wait until the damage is severe, it could be costly and inconvenient to fix.

Why not spend a little time each day stopping this awful disease from growing and causing further damage? It just plain makes sense to do so. Or, if you have not developed that severe of a condition yet, why not just work on preventing it now?

There are a lot of misconceptions about gingivitis. I heard one older gentleman remark, "I'm getting old, so of course my gums are going to recede." I say that is not necessarily the case. If this gentleman did the same basic work that a person of any other age can do, he should expect similar results. That is not to say that age is not a factor. But gum disease and receding gums take time to develop. They do not normally happen overnight.

If your gums bleed when you brush or floss your teeth, there is a very good chance that you have gum disease or the beginnings of it. It is really not normal for healthy gum tissue to bleed. The gum tissue, when healthy, is fairly resilient.

The major problem with gum disease is that it can cause you to lose your teeth. In fact, it is the number one cause of tooth loss. Many people might think that cavities would be the number one cause, but that is not the case. Gum disease is.

The same older gentleman I just mentioned also said there is no substitute for having your own, real teeth. And he is right. Nature knows best what works for us and no artificial substitute is going to be completely up to par.

If you have gum disease or gingivitis, please contact your dentist for diagnosis and treatment.

David Snape is the author of the book, *What You Should Know about Gum Disease*. You can find Dave and ask him questions about gum disease or other health, fitness, or wellness topics at: http://whatyoushouldknowaboutgumdisease.com

Do You Have Gum Disease?

Gum disease has been deemed a silent epidemic. It can rob a person of his teeth. But how much do you really know about this disease? Can it be stopped or prevented? I believe the answer is yes in many cases, but not all.

Most people are woefully unaware they even have gum disease, that is, until the situation becomes critical. So, how do you know if you have gum disease? The best way to be sure is to get a diagnosis from your dentist or, even better, a periodontist.

However, if your gums bleed upon brushing or flossing, there is a good possibility that you have gum disease. Some people do not care if they have it or not. I think they would care if they lost some or all of their teeth. Who would want to deal with dentures or implants if they did not have to?

I spoke to a dental student recently and she told me that people actually come to the clinic and ask for all of their teeth to be pulled. They do not want to spend the time it takes to clean them properly. The problem is that even if someone has that done, they still have to take care of the dentures, and the gum tissue around implants still needs to be cared for. So, not much is resolved by having all of one's teeth pulled.

There is a rare two percent of the population that is virtually immune to gum disease. If true, that would mean that the other ninety-eight percent of us are prone. Official quotes say that something like seventy-five percent of people over the age of

191

thirty-five have gingivitis or gum disease. My guess is that the number may be higher.

Wouldn't it be wonderful if there was a fairly simple solution to get rid of gum disease? Let me tell you my story. One day, seemingly out of the blue, my hygienist wanted me to sign a paper that stated it was not the dental office's fault if I lost my teeth. I was a little shocked. But the truth is, this situation did not develop overnight. Just like I mentioned before, it took years for gum disease to progress to that point.

I did not know that a little occasional bleeding while brushing or flossing was not normal. In fact, many people are unaware. The truth is that it is not considered normal for your gums to bleed while brushing or flossing.

Once I did my research, I found a few simple tools that helped me to eliminate the problem. When I went back to the dentist's office, they were amazed. The last time I went, the hygienist said that there was no bleeding during probing. That is a good sign for the health of my gums.

If you have or think you might have something as serious as gum disease, visit your dentist for diagnosis and treatment. Stop gum disease and keep your teeth for the long haul.

David Snape is the author of the book, *What You Should Know about Gum Disease*. You can find Dave and ask him questions about gum disease or other health, fitness, or wellness topics at: http://whatyoushouldknowaboutgumdisease.com. David also practices the easy, gentle but powerful exercises of Falun Dafa.

You can learn more about them at the FalunDafa.org website.

My Gums are Bleeding—What Should I Do?

I recently heard from a woman who told me that her gums bled frequently. She said that she has blood in her mouth when she wakes up in the morning. She also said she could not afford to go to the dentist.

I told her that she must go. Chances are she has gum disease, but she needs a dentist or doctor to diagnose the situation and rule out anything more serious.

This brings up an important point. Bleeding gums are not normal at all. Usually, if your gums bleed while brushing or flossing it is probably indicative of gum disease.

Here is a quote from the Food and Drug Administration's website:

> "More than 75 percent of Americans over 35 have some form of gum disease. In its earliest stage, your gums might swell and bleed easily. At its worst, you might lose your teeth. The bottom-line? If you want to keep your teeth, you must take care of your gums."

Isn't that scary? But it underscores a point. Gum disease or gingivitis is serious. Not only can you lose your teeth, but with gum disease you also have what amounts to open wounds in your mouth. Those crazy little bacteria might find their way into the bloodstream via those openings. Whether that situation can lead to something worse or not is still being studied. This is what the FDA has to say about that:

> "[The] CDC cautions that there is not enough evidence to conclude that oral infections actually cause or contribute to cardiovascular disease, diabetes and other serious

health problems. More research is underway to determine whether the associations are causal or coincidental."

In any case, the possibility of losing one's teeth is real. And that is a situation that should be avoided.

In my personal experience, I was the patient of the same dentist for years. I knew my gums bled during those every-six-month cleanings, but I did not know that meant I had gum disease. They did not tell me that. I thought it was normal, as do a lot of people. Then one day they suggested that I get a scaling and root planing. They also told me that I had lost bone mass and that if things progressed I could lose my teeth.

Fortunately, I had enough sense to do a little research. I found a solution that really worked. I know it worked because the next time I visited, they told me how much healthier my gums were looking and that I no longer needed the scaling and root planing.

In that procedure, they dig under the gum line and scrape away the tartar or plaque that has built up. They feel that this buildup is responsible for making the gum tissue pull away from the tooth, ultimately leading to the loss of gum tissue and the supporting bone structure.

I did not want the expense, pain, or hassle of going through such a procedure. And I also know someone who had that procedure done and she has expressed to me more than once that it was not worthwhile.

I like my teeth and felt that this was an important enough situation that I needed to understand exactly what was going on. My personal philosophy is that I like to know as much as possible about any health condition or procedure before allowing anything to be done. Knowledge is power, so they say.

If you have gingivitis, gum disease, or think you might, go to your dentist right away for diagnosis and treatment. Keeping your teeth is important. Getting rid of gum disease is desirable.

David Snape is the author of the book, *What You Should Know about Gum Disease*. You can find Dave and ask him questions about gum disease or other health, fitness, or wellness topics at:
http://whatyoushouldknowaboutgumdisease.com.

Gum Disease is Underestimated

My personal experience with gum disease motivated me to discover a way to fight it without expensive treatments. I found that gum disease is a very common problem, not only in humans, but also in domesticated pets.

Did you know that most people are likely to experience gingivitis or gum disease at some point in their lives? This makes sense when you really think about it. The mouth becomes really dirty from eating. It is not easy to keep your teeth and gums clean. Only about two percent of people seem to have a natural immunity to gum disease.

If you look at your mouth carefully after a meal, you will see exactly what I mean. You could notice food stuck in your teeth and mashed up against the gums. This debris needs to be routinely removed from the mouth. Brushing and flossing alone are not necessarily enough to keep plaque from forming.

Plaque is a nasty, thin, sticky film that allows anaerobic bacteria to be trapped between itself and the hard surface of your tooth. In this environment, the bacteria can thrive. If the plaque hardens into tartar, it provides an even better place for these bacteria to live and begin the process of destroying both teeth and gums. Therefore, it is important to make sure that this layer of plaque does not get to develop.

Some say that once tartar forms, the only way to get it off is via a professional dental cleaning. The rate of tartar formation varies from one person to another. It can form fairly quickly in some people and less so in others.

Frankly, gum disease is a terrible thing when you really think about it. If allowed to progress, it can cause a person to lose his/her teeth. Depending on whom you believe, the problems might not stop there. The presence of gum disease could also allow bacteria to invade the blood stream and contribute to a number of diseases. There is still debate, but there are credentialed professionals who believe this to be true. The founder of a popular clinic said that the loss of a person's teeth could take ten years off one's life span.

Generally speaking, the public is not well educated about gum disease, what it can do and how serious it is. Often times, people do not become aware of the disease until bone and tissue loss have already occurred. By then, it might be time for expensive treatments to correct the damage.

Why let things get to that point? As the saying goes, "An ounce of prevention is worth a pound of cure." Become educated about this "silent epidemic," and take steps to protect yourself and your family.

If you have or think you have gum disease, gingivitis, or any other health problem, be sure to visit your dentist or doctor for diagnosis and treatment.

David Snape is the author of the book, *What You Should Know about Gum Disease*. You can find Dave and ask questions about gum disease or other health, fitness, or wellness topics at: http://whatyoushouldknowaboutgumdisease.com.

Fighting Gum Disease with the Hydro Floss

Have you ever attempted to remove a screw without a screwdriver? Maybe you have tried to collect leaves without a rake, or change a car's tire with a less-than-adequate jack? Without the right tools, it can be really hard to get a job done properly and efficiently. It might even be impossible to do the job at all.

When it comes to oral health and fighting gum disease, the same concept applies. Manually brushing and flossing are not always potent enough for preventing gum disease, and are perhaps even less sufficient for stopping an existing case. However, brushing and flossing can help and are still very important for oral health.

I was told at my dentist's office that I had lost some of the bone structure supporting my teeth due to moderate gum disease. This was shocking to me because I did not know I had gum disease in the first place.

Like many people, I thought that it was no big deal if my gums bled slightly when brushing or flossing. I was certainly wrong about that. Bleeding gums, even a little bit, is a prime sign of gum disease.

I was told that I needed a special treatment. They wanted to dig under my gums to get rid of built up tartar and plaque. That sounded both painful and expensive to me. Worse, they wanted to start immediately.

There was not much time to think. I decided that I would hold off on the treatment and do a little research on my own. One of the major dangers of having gum disease is that you can lose your teeth. Therefore, I was highly motivated to find answers that made sense to me.

In the process of my research, I stumbled across the Hydro Floss. I decided to get one and see what kind of results I could obtain. I found that the Hydro Floss is a wonderful tool for cleaning around the neck of the teeth where the gum line is.

Using the Hydro Floss was a major step towards progress. On its own, however, it did not seem like it was enough to completely change the health of my gum tissue. So I added another item to the mix.

Between these two tools, I have found a method that allowed me to stop the progression of gum disease and prevent its return. The proof came when I returned to the dentist's office. I was told that I no longer needed the root scaling and planing. The tarter buildup was no longer below the gum line.

On subsequent visits, it was clear that my gum tissue was getting healthier and healthier. I do not have bleeding anymore, even when the hygienist uses a metal probe to check the health of my gums.

You could say that I am absolutely delighted at the results!

David Snape is the author of the book, *What You Should Know about Gum Disease*. You can find Dave and ask questions about gum disease or other health, fitness, or wellness topics at: http://whatyoushouldknowaboutgumdisease.com. You can find a Hydro Floss oral irrigator at http://tobeinformed.com/421

Gingivitis and Gum Disease Can Be Prevented

They wanted me to submit to a scaling and root planing procedure. They said it would not hurt because they would numb my gums before proceeding. Did I want to get started today?

NO! I did NOT want to start today. I wondered why I needed this procedure all of a sudden!

As I looked further into the situation, a larger picture began to reveal itself. It became apparent that I was the victim of gum disease, the silent epidemic that stalks most people who do not usually realize it until it is time for a costly and potentially painful treatment and recovery.

What I think is disturbing is that a condition does not get this bad between office visits. Why did I suddenly need this treatment? Why wasn't this mentioned before? How come I was not told how to prevent it? In fact, gum disease often develops slowly over a period of years. More importantly, it is preventable.

Gum recession and tissue that is lost will not normally return completely. Some gum recession can remain even if you go to a periodontist, who can rebuild some tissue by inserting bone matrix or by utilizing other similar procedures. This is also an expensive proposition.

As I mentioned before, I declined the scaling and root planing. The response from the hygienist was that she wanted me to sign a paper that it was not their fault if I lost my teeth. My satisfaction came six months later when the hygienist looked at my mouth and said that I did not need that scaling and root planing any longer.

My frustration, however, lingers. I had visited the same dentist's office for about eight years. This did not happen overnight. Why wasn't I ever told how to stop gum disease from getting worse? Going back even further, why was I not told how to prevent it? The gum recession does not reverse by itself. The gums might be healthy again, but the tissue loss remains.

Here is a quote from the Mayo Clinic website: "Nearly 80 percent of American adults have some form of gum (periodontal) disease." The question that begs to be answered is: How do I prevent this in the first place?

Unfortunately, you could get an answer suggesting that brushing and flossing are important. I agree they are important, but it is difficult to believe that eighty percent of Americans are not brushing and flossing. Just thinking about the numbers leads to the conclusion that brushing and flossing are NOT enough to prevent gum disease for most people.

I found a combination of materials that I could use to stop gum disease from getting worse. It was a great discovery for me, personally. The last time I visited the dentist, there was no bleeding. My gums are a healthy pink now. Unfortunately, getting the lost tissue back would involve some expensive treatment and potentially painful recovery time.

Fortunately, I can prevent further problems. I wish that I had an article like this one in my hands fifteen years ago. That way, I could have kept the gum tissue that I had. My teeth and gums look fine, even when I smile. It's when I look closely that I notice just how much tissue was lost. It did not have to be that way. If things had gotten worse, I could have lost teeth over this disease. Do not lose yours. If you have gum disease or suspect you might, visit your dentist for diagnosis and treatment.

David Snape is the author of the book, *What You Should Know about Gum Disease.* You can find Dave and ask questions about gum disease or other health, fitness, or wellness topics at: http://whatyoushouldknowaboutgumdisease.com.

How Did I Get Gum Disease?

Gum disease afflicts up to eighty percent of Americans, according to statistics. Just imagine, eight out of ten of the people you personally know could already have gum disease. This is a problem that can lead to tooth loss. Some believe that gum disease also leads to more serious health conditions as it creates a pathway for bacteria to enter the body.

Know anyone who has returned from the dentist's office after being told that he needed a scaling and root planing or needed to see a periodontist because he had gum disease? This scenario plays itself out in dentists' offices frequently.

What is going on?

Why does someone suddenly get gum disease? The answer is that one probably did not *suddenly* get it. Chances are, it has been working its evil quietly in that person's life for a really long time. This person has been getting "long in the tooth" for many years now. This is gum recession and it goes hand-in-hand with gum disease.

But why weren't you told about it before?

Now that I have been paying attention to the health of people's gums when they speak, I can often see red puffy gums in even young twenty-something-year-olds. I have read from a dentist who states that perhaps somewhere between seventy-five and ninety-five percent of people have gum disease. Why?

Even for people who take scrupulously good care of their teeth by brushing and flossing daily, many will still develop gum disease.

Why is this happening?

Consider the nature of eating. Our teeth are designed to mash and crush food during the process of mastication (eating). All that force being applied to mash our food into digestible, tiny pieces is likely to squeeze many food particles against our teeth and gums. A substance called plaque may begin to form. Plaque provides a nifty anaerobic environment for bacteria that cause gum disease to live, grow, and reproduce in.

Plaque can harden into a substance called tartar. Tartar provides an even better environment for bacteria to thrive in.

Brushing and flossing are not always enough to prevent plaque or tartar from forming. Removing tartar proves to be even more difficult. Many dental professionals say that tartar can only be removed via a professional cleaning. This could very well be part of the reason that the Mayo Clinic's website says up to eighty percent of Americans have this disease.

When I found out that I needed a scaling and root planing, I was a bit unhappy. I knew that this condition did not develop overnight. I was disappointed that I was never taught prevention. I have found that patient education on prevention has been a bit lacking, at least among the dentists that I have visited.

I declined the scaling and root planing that was offered to me.

Instead, I decided to research what was happening. I discovered a combination of tools that helped me to stop the gum disease I was suffering from. After returning to the dentist's office, I was told that I no longer needed that scaling and root planing treatment. I am delighted at the results I have obtained.

I might not be able to get the gum tissue that I lost to return. But I can take steps to prevent gum disease from coming back and work to preserve the gum tissue that I have left. If you have or think you might have gum disease, you should visit a dentist for diagnosis and treatment.

David Snape is the author of the book, *What You Should Know about Gum Disease*. You can find Dave and ask questions about gum disease or other health, fitness, or wellness topics at:

http://whatyoushouldknowaboutgumdisease.com.

An Alternative to Scaling and Root Planing Worked For Me

Recently, I was looking at some "official" information about gum disease and gingivitis. One of the sites implied that gum disease was the result of poor brushing and flossing habits. I think this is possibly an untrue and potentially dangerous statement to make because it could lead people to believe they will be safe from gum disease if they brush and floss regularly.

The Mayo Clinic's website estimates that about eighty percent of Americans suffer from gum disease. Another source states that between seventy-five and ninety-five percent of the population is affected. If someone were to suggest that eighty percent of Americans do not brush or floss properly, my response would be that although many Americans might have this problem, it is not very likely that eighty percent do. I think it is more plausible to conclude that brushing and flossing are generally not enough to prevent gum disease.

In my own example, I brushed and flossed, likely more frequently than the average person, and still developed gum disease. I visited a hygienist's website and she wrote that regular brushing and flossing were not enough to prevent gum disease. With decades of experience backing her up, I think her opinion is a qualified one.

Age is not likely to be a determining factor, either. I have noticed that even some very young adults have red or purplish swollen gums. This is sad. I am positive that the dental profession could create new excellent and effective home regimens that would help the vast majority of adults avoid gum disease or defeat it. If you are a dentist reading this, I hope that you will personally take up the banner of preventing gum disease and champion this cause.

Yes, one day, I was told that I needed a scaling and root planing, and I was quite surprised. I did not really understand what gum disease was and did not believe that I actually had it. I thought it was normal for some bleeding to occur during brushing and flossing. I later discovered that notion was incorrect. Bleeding during brushing and flossing is a symptom of gum disease. If the gums bleed while brushing or flossing—even a little bit—it is NOT normal.

A relative told me that she had a scaling and root planing treatment done, that the results were not good, and that she felt her gums were worse than before the treatment. I elected not to have the treatment done and decided to do my own research. What I found was quite alarming. The number one cause of tooth loss is gum disease. More people have it (or its precursor, gingivitis), than you might reasonably suspect.

I was still puzzled by the question of what to do about it. Then, I stumbled upon a few things that, in combination, worked to improve the health of my gums. As a result, on my very next office visit I was told that my gums were looking better, and that I did not need that root scaling and planing treatment because they were not detecting tartar under the gum line.

If you have or think you might have gum disease or gingivitis, visit your dentist right away for diagnosis and treatment.

David Snape is the author of the book, *What You Should Know about Gum Disease*. You can find Dave and ask questions about gum disease or other health, fitness, or wellness topics at: http://whatyoushouldknowaboutgumdisease.com.

Beware of Gum Disease

The silent epidemic called gum disease rages on around the world just as it has for centuries. It has been on a never-ending rampage for thousands of years. "So what?" you might think. Considering that gum disease is the number one cause of tooth loss, someone with it is probably going to care sooner or later.

Gum disease affects nearly eighty percent of adult Americans, according to a popular clinic's website. Some estimate the number to be even higher. If eighty percent of the population is afflicted, then most of your friends have it, and the odds say you do, too. Yet, you or others who are afflicted with gum disease probably do not even know it. Age is no protection either—gum disease can exist in children as young as six years old!

Can gum disease be prevented or stopped? Most professionals believe it can be with excellent oral hygiene. But what does it mean to have excellent hygiene? If you do not spend excessive amounts of time cleaning your teeth and gums multiple times a day, what is the solution?

I am of the opinion that brushing and flossing alone are not enough to stop or prevent gum disease. Actually, I would venture to guess that more than twenty percent of the adult American population brush and floss daily. Therefore, I would conclude that brushing and flossing must not be enough to prevent gum disease or stop its development.

Given the modern technology that we have, there should be more powerful tools with which to fight gum disease. The Hydro Floss is a powerful oral irrigator that can help you clean around and just below the gum line. Yet, I found that even when using such a device, the fight against gum disease was a slow and painful process. That is, until I found additional products, tools, and techniques to give gum disease the knockout punch from home.

However, there is not much that I can do for the bone and tissue loss that has already occurred. If I had understood prevention a little better, I could have stopped or mitigated the amount of tissue and bone loss I did suffer. Like many people, I did not realize that I actually had gum disease until the tissue and bone had been lost.

I still have all of my teeth, and enough gum tissue and supporting bone structure left to have a natural smile. I am just pointing out that had I been doing earlier what I am currently doing, I would be a little bit less "long in the tooth" now.

Today, even lost gum tissue and supporting bone structure can be replaced, but the expense can be rather high and the results not what were hoped for. Technology is still limited in this regard. If the recession is large scale, it might not be possible to do much. Why let it get that way in the first place? Why risk the loss of a tooth or multiple teeth? Discover what you can do to stop the progression of gum disease and prevent its return.

Visit your dentist for diagnosis and treatment if you have or think you might have gum disease.

David Snape is the author of the book, *What You Should Know about Gum Disease.* You can find Dave and ask questions about gum disease or other health, fitness, or wellness topics at: http://whatyoushouldknowaboutgumdisease.com.

Gum Disease Alternative

Prevention is the best alternative to expensive gum surgery treatments. These treatments are costly and several could be needed depending on the degree of the problem. However, even when the surgery is over, you still need to prevent a recurrence. In addition, the surgery might not be able to return all of the gum tissue you have lost.

If you already suffer from gum disease, now is the time to start fighting it. If you are able to stop its progression, you will then want to focus on preventing a recurrence. Most have the ability to do this.

Even when you think you have made progress against gum disease, if the supporting tissue is lost, there could come a day when a toothbrush or food particle irritates the gums to the point that the unsupported tissue recedes, exposing more of the tooth root. Once bone and tissue loss occurs to a certain degree, it can be a struggle to save one's teeth; surgery could even be necessary.

An ounce of prevention is worth a pound of cure, as the saying goes. Estimates from a popular clinic are that eighty percent of American adults have gum disease. So are brushing and flossing enough to prevent gum disease, then? When contemplating that statistic, it does not seem very likely.

Do all the possible research you can before you even start to encounter any gingivitis. It is so very important to understand what this insidious disease can do. Next, you need to be able to recognize it. Do not make the mistake I made. I thought it was normal for my gums to bleed occasionally while brushing or flossing. Unfortunately, I had no idea that bleeding is not normal at all.

When tartar and plaque build up under the gum line, you are in trouble. So do not let it happen in the first place. Gum disease is the number one cause of tooth loss. If you want to keep all of your teeth, learn about prevention early. Even if you already have gum disease, you should learn about every possible thing you could do to arrest its progress.

Gum disease and gingivitis are far more serious than you probably imagine. Gum recession, bone loss, and possible tooth loss can occur. When gum disease develops momentum, your options could be limited. Expensive and multiple surgeries could be needed to save your gums and teeth, and there is no guarantee after all that work, either.

Research indicates that gum disease possibly contributes to heart disease, stroke, and other illnesses. The jury is still out deciding this matter and not everyone is convinced. Why take any chances?

If you already have gum disease, find out what you can do to fight it. If you do not have it yet, start working to prevent it now. Teach your children well so that they can preserve their gums and teeth for a lifetime of use. If you have, or think you have, gum disease, be sure to visit your dentist for diagnosis and treatment.

David Snape is the author of the book, *What You Should Know about Gum Disease*. You can find Dave and ask questions about gum disease or other health, fitness, or wellness topics at: http://whatyoushouldknowaboutgumdisease.com.

Gum Disease Requires Immediate Action

A sad fact about human nature exists that few of us—if any—can escape; we like to procrastinate. We procrastinate both collectively and as individuals.

Have you ever noticed that people will not join together to accomplish something unless there is a strong and underlying driving force causing a need? For example, Americans banded together in a spirit of cooperation and patriotism for WWII.

When it comes to individuals working on their own, it is a bit more difficult. Becoming and staying motivated is a state that is hard to produce at will. I'm sure you know exactly what I mean and have multiple examples of your own.

We will typically get motivated when we have an overwhelming drive and multiple deep-set reasons to accomplish a goal. If that fundamental base is not in place, it will be a long uphill battle to get yourself or others to do something that requires sustained effort.

So how does this factor into fighting or preventing gum disease? Both require a lot of hard work. If you already have gum disease, you will have to put in some effort to stop its progression. You will also have to work hard to keep it from coming back.

Part of the motivation to overcome these obstacles should be the desire to save one's teeth. Gum disease is the number one cause of tooth loss. Preventing or fighting an existing case of gum disease is really the battle to save one's teeth. Some people talk about gum disease as providing a pathway into the body for bacteria to cause further health problems.

Does the kind of prevention we are referring to involve brushing and flossing? They are important activities, to be sure; but are they enough to stop gum disease from getting a foothold? The Mayo Clinic website says that up to eighty percent of adult Americans have gum disease.

The numbers are probably equally high in other nations. In America, we are obsessed with caring for our teeth. Still, so many people are afflicted. If brushing and flossing were enough to prevent gum disease for most people, the Mayo statistic would have to be much lower.

So, we have to be motivated to do the right things after finding out what they are. One of the problems is finding decent information along with the right tools and the knowledge of what to do with them.

I was told that I had gum disease. However, I was not told what I could personally do about it. Instead, the dentist gave me a treatment option that did not sound palatable to me. I needed to do some research and see if there was some kind of home care that would be easier and more convenient to use. I was able to find a combination of tools that allowed me to check the progression of gum disease and prevent its return.

Get motivated. If you know you have gum disease, take action right away. Measured by time, money, and aggravation, treatments become more costly as conditions worsen. Visit your dentist for diagnosis and treatment if you have or think you might have gum disease or gingivitis.

David Snape is the author of the book, *What You Should Know about Gum Disease.* You can find Dave and ask questions about gum disease or other health, fitness, or wellness topics at: http://whatyoushouldknowaboutgumdisease.com.

Periodontitis Risk Factors

Periodontitis is an inflammation of the bone, gums and supporting structure of the teeth. It is a bacterial infection that afflicts the tissue around and supporting a tooth's root. Periodontitis is gum disease.

Most professionals agree that gum disease can be prevented. They often refer to good oral hygiene habits as the key to preventing gum disease. I agree. However, what does good oral hygiene constitute? Some say that brushing, flossing, and having professional cleanings done once every six months is enough to prevent gum disease. Yet seventy-five percent of Americans over the age of thirty-five have gum disease, and sixty percent of those know little or nothing about gum disease.

Perhaps the professionals who take care of our teeth and gums could improve patient education. Could it be that regular brushing and flossing, as well as every-six-month professional cleanings, might not be enough to prevent gum disease in everyone after all? Discerning the truth of the matter is difficult.

What kind of risk factors potentially contribute to the likelihood of periodontitis developing in your mouth? There are several. These factors were noted on the FDA's website.

- **Smoking:** People who smoke are seven times more likely to develop periodontitis than people who do not smoke. Smoking is bad for virtually every part of our bodies and our gum tissue health is also affected by it. The increased risk for gum disease is yet one more reason to quit now.

- **Hormonal Changes:** Hormones appear to have a major impact on the health of our gums. You have probably heard the term "pregnancy gingivitis" before. Though a person can be more susceptible to this disease, it might still be preventable. Gum disease should not be considered inevitable for all people.

- **Stress:** Stress limits the body's ability to fight off disease. There is no surprise there.

- **Medication:** A side effect to certain medications is to decrease the flow of saliva. Saliva is helpful in protecting the health of both the teeth and the gums. Other drugs, like diphenylhydantoin (for convulsions) and nifedipine (for angina), can cause abnormal growth of gum tissue. Those are just examples and there are plenty of other medications out there. Ask your pharmacist specifically about the medication you are, or will be taking.

- **Poor Nutrition:** Not getting the right nutrients to keep the body healthy can contribute to the progression of many diseases indirectly, and sometimes directly. This has to do with giving the body the nutrients it needs to repair itself properly, as well as promoting a strong immune system. *You are what you eat*, as the saying goes. Eating sugar will increase the acidity of the mouth, which often creates a better environment for bacteria to live in.

- **Illnesses:** Illness may interfere with your body's ability to fight off additional infection, including the kind that leads to gum disease.

- **Grinding Teeth:** This often happens when we are sleeping. I know I have this problem and I try to wear a dental guard. These guards can be obtained at virtually any drug store. However, long term use of that variety is not recommended. Getting a custom guard made by your dentist would be a better idea.

If you have or think you might have gum disease, gingivitis, or any other oral health condition, contact your dentist or periodontist for diagnosis and treatment.

David Snape is the author of the book, *What You Should Know about Gum Disease.* You can find Dave and ask questions about gum disease or other health, fitness, or wellness topics at: http://whatyoushouldknowaboutgumdisease.com.

Gum Disease and Your Genes
In November of 2000, the *Journal of Clinical Periodontology* published a study about gum disease and genetics. Using identical twins as test subjects, it was determined that genetics play a role in a person's susceptibility to gum disease.

Since the Mayo Clinic's website mentions that about eighty percent of adult Americans have some form of gum disease, a genetic predisposition could mean that such a person has to be extra careful to prevent gum disease, and ever more diligent to fight off an existing case. If one or both of your parents have lost teeth due to gum disease, you are probably more likely than average to contract the disease. On the other side of the spectrum, about two percent of the population seems to have a natural immunity to gum disease. That leaves about ninety-eight percent of us who need to be concerned about prevention or stopping the progression of it.

Bacterial toxins irritate the gingiva or gum tissue and cause gum disease. The constant assault upon your gum tissue can even harm the bone structure underneath. That structure is what supports the gums and teeth. As a result, the teeth can become loose and even fall out.

Being young is not necessarily going to preclude one from contracting gum disease. In fact, bacterial infection of the gingiva has been noted in children as young as six years old!

So what can you do? Proper brushing and flossing are certainly helpful, but if the Mayo Clinic statistic is correct, that is possibly not enough. What does it mean to brush and floss correctly, anyway? Certainly, this is an excellent question for your dentist or hygienist. I have also formed my own ideas in this area. Not all dental professionals agree that regular brushing and flossing are enough to prevent gingivitis or gum disease, or eliminate them once they have occurred. In any case, brushing and flossing are still useful measures and should not be abandoned. And for some, they are possibly all that is needed. I do not offer much on exactly how I use a toothbrush because I think it is very important to follow the advice of your periodontist or hygienist.

Irrigating with a device designed to shoot a stream of water around the gum line, thereby cleaning that area, is an excellent practice in addition to brushing and flossing. Personally, I have made one additional step and added something that has helped me tremendously in the fight against gum disease.

The outcome of this experiment on my part was being told that I no longer needed a special gum treatment (root scaling and planing treatment). Furthermore, I was told there was no bleeding on a subsequent checkup. Bleeding during probing points to the existence of gum disease. I used to have a great deal of bleeding when they cleaned my teeth or probed my gums with dental instruments.

Try to avoid the mistake of thinking you do not have gum disease. Remember the Mayo Clinic statistic. Those stats show that most people have it. If you do not, you are probably the exception rather than the rule. Specifically ask your dentist and hygienist each time you go in for a checkup if you have gum disease and to what degree. They should be telling you the amount of pocket depth for the gum tissue around each tooth each time you visit. Anything over 3mm of pocket depth is considered abnormal. Those are areas you should pay special attention to. Have your hygienist point out the danger areas where plaque and tartar tend to accumulate in your mouth between visits. Then give those areas special focus at home.

If you have, or think you might have, gum disease, contact your dentist for diagnosis and treatment.

David Snape is the author of the book, *What You Should Know about Gum Disease.* You can find Dave and ask questions about gum disease or other health, fitness, or wellness topics, at: http://whatyoushould-knowaboutgumdisease.com. The cornerstone of his personal, overall health regimen is the practice of Falun Dafa. You can read about the peaceful, energizing exercises on the FalunDafa.org website.

Reversible Pulpitis
The words hung in the air and the implied meaning struck me like a hammer. There was no way I was going to allow this dentist to make

a permanent hole in my tooth and then fill it after hearing the word *reversible*. I was going to do a little research first. I feared that what the dentist wanted to do and what was really necessary were two very divergent realities. It turns out I was right.

I did my research. The majority of the sources I checked indicated that reversible pulpitis will go away without intervention. Why then did this dentist want to drill into my perfectly good tooth? That is a question that still disturbs me, more than a year later.

It does appear that there is a gray area nestled in among the qualified opinions of dentists. Some believe that the very beginning of tooth decay should be immediately drilled and filled. Others are not so quick on the draw.

Having a number of negative experiences with dentists, I have become a bit cautious around them. It should be pointed out that there are plenty of very good, ethical, and well-intentioned dentists. I just tend to lean a bit more on the side of caution and conservative treatment. It has paid off on at least a couple of occasions to hold off on immediate treatment and do a little research first.

I equate the dentist's attempt to start right away, with the type of high-pressure tactics that often take place on a used car lot. The stakes are a little higher in the former case. The health of our teeth and gum tissue is not the realm where sharp salesmen or NLP-wielding marketers should tread. Yet, the phrase, "Let the buyer beware," still seems apropos.

What happened at the end of my story? I dropped that dentist like a bad habit. I was so sure that nothing was wrong that I did not even bother getting a second opinion. Six months later, I went to another dentist, and guess what? There was no cavity in sight. "But, isn't it in my chart?" I asked. "Yes, I see it in there." Not wanting to harm the reputation of the other dentist, I decided not to say anymore.

I have thought a lot about it, though. The words that first dentist said before declaring her wish to drill and fill my tooth were about her impending wedding. I cannot help but think she felt some special need to make more money than her usual take.

I briefly considered reporting her to the state board that regulates her profession. I decided not to. I believe in the saying, "What goes around comes around." I do not wish for anything bad to happen to this dentist. I just believe there is a universal justice system that balances things out in the end.

In any case, I am glad I did not have a cavity that was permanent. The moral of this story underscores a point I think is important. The body does have the ability to heal itself. Softness in dental enamel is no different. Still, perhaps there are times when it cannot. Once it crosses the threshold between reversible and irreversible pulpitis, then you really do have a cavity that needs to be filled.

Of course, I am not a dentist and I am not suggesting self-diagnosis or treatment. If you have, or think you might have, a cavity or any other dental condition, you should go to your dentist for diagnosis and treatment.

Apparently you can sometimes start to develop a cavity and it can go away. I found a reference to a November 1991 study published in the *Journal of Oral Rehabilitation* in PubMed. (PMID 1762023). The Dental Research Unit of Hadassah Medical School located in Jerusalem, Israel conducted this study.

After intentionally softening enamel utilizing a popular cola drink, they found significant hardening of the enamel from eating hard cheese. This is important because it suggests that when the tooth enamel is weakened, it can become strong again.

This makes sense because the human body is not a machine in the true sense. For example, a car does not have any self-healing mechanisms. It breaks down sooner than a human body and requires external intervention to keep it running. The human body has many ways to heal itself. Consider a cut or an abrasion and how the body can often repair those problems without medical intervention.

Remember, if you have or think you might have any dental problems or other health problems at all, be sure to consult your dentist or doctor for advice, diagnosis, and treatment.

David Snape is the author of the book, *What You Should Know about Gum Disease.* You can find Dave and ask questions about gum disease or other health, fitness, or wellness topics at: http://whatyoushouldknowaboutgumdisease.com. The cornerstone of his personal health maintenance regimen comprises the peaceful exercises of Falun Dafa. You can read and watch videos about them on the http://www.FalunDafa.org website.

Gum Disease Risk Factors

Gum disease is a widespread but silent problem. Many people do not understand the seriousness of this insidious epidemic until their smiles become less attractive and their gums have receded. If that doesn't draw a person's attention to the situation, loose and lost teeth will.

Unfortunately, this is what it sometimes takes for a person to sit up and take notice. It is hard to be on guard against something if you do not recognize it as a problem. That is just human nature and is understandable. However, "An ounce of prevention is worth a pound of cure," as the saying goes. If you do not think gum disease or gingivitis is something you need to worry about, the odds state otherwise. The Mayo Clinic website estimates that about eighty percent of adult Americans have some form of this disease.

Eight out of ten adults is quite a large number of people. So this is something that the majority of people need to be concerned about. Here are some specific factors that can contribute to the development or intensity of an existing gum disease problem.

1. **Smoking**—Smoking harms most of the body's tissues and immune system. You need a fairly strong immune system to combat gum disease. If you smoke or chew tobacco, you should probably stop. This is just one more from a long list of reasons to quit the use of cigarettes and chewing tobacco.

2. **Clenching or Grinding the Teeth**—This is a big one for some people. If you grind your teeth, you probably should get a mouth guard, which can be bought at most any drug store. Ask someone if they hear you grinding your teeth while you sleep. The extreme pressures generated from clenching and grinding can weaken the supporting structure of your teeth and gums. This can make it easier for a gum tissue infection to occur, or increase the progression of an existing invasion.

3. **Medications**—Certain medications can affect the health of the gum tissue. Whenever you pick up a medication from your local pharmacy, you should ask the pharmacist for a print out of side effects. This will be quite an eye opener to you. Look for any side effect that mentions oral

health, drying of the mouth, periodontitis, or gum disease in particular.

4. **Pregnancy and Hormones**—Hormonal changes can affect your gums. In addition, a woman with an existing case of gum disease could be up to seven times more likely to have a low birth weight, preterm child.

5. **Genetics**—Studies done on identical twins seem to indicate that there is a genetic factor that comes into play with gum disease. Some people are more susceptible and have to work harder to prevent plaque buildup on their teeth, especially near the gums. On the other end of the spectrum, apparently two percent of the population is resistant to gum disease. This shows that what genes you inherit can have an impact on your oral health.

7. **Stress**—Stress affects the immune system of the body. A healthy immune system is important in fighting off infections, including the bacteria that cause gum disease. Too much stress weakens the immune system.

8. **Diabetes**—In general, those who suffer from diabetes are at higher risk to contract infections. Gum disease is an infection of the gum tissue. This is also true for any other disease that affects or compromises the immune system.

Gum disease is fairly common, and even if you think you do not have it, you very well could. Ask your dentist at every checkup if you are showing any signs of gum disease. Develop superior oral care habits now and you could keep your teeth and gums healthy for the rest of your life.

If you already have gum disease, now is a good time to take action. In addition to checking with your dentist for diagnosis and treatment, research everything you can about gum disease. Before trying any alternative methods or treatments, be sure to consult with your dentist.

David Snape is the author of the book, *What You Should Know about Gum Disease.* You can find Dave and ask questions about gum disease or other health, fitness, or wellness topics at: http://whatyoushouldknowaboutgumdisease.com. Dave also practices the very gentle but powerful exercises of Falun Dafa. You can find them described in detail and even watch video instructions at the http://FalunDafa.org/ website.

Gum Disease and Plaque

A widely held belief is that the bacteria that live in the plaque on your teeth—and near or under your gums—is responsible for creating gum disease. This plaque is constantly forming and must constantly be removed or it will accumulate to the detriment of our gums and teeth. Once formed, anaerobic bacteria will grow under it and secrete harmful toxins that attack our gum tissue and the tooth's supporting structure.

For all practical purposes, gum disease is a chronic disease. The body has defenses that can slow the progression of gum disease and loss of gum tissue, but in most cases, those defenses do not seem to be enough to eradicate progression completely by itself. This necessitates the need for both excellent home care habits and professional care with a regular dental cleaning schedule.

When the problems progress beyond a certain point, dentists and periodontists have specialized surgical and nonsurgical treatments to help, but in about twenty percent of the population, these treatments will do little to change the long-term health of the gums. (Reference: Clin Microbial Rev. 2001 October; 14(4): 727–752. doi: 10.1128/CMR.14.4.727-752.2001. — "...current standard of care, i.e., the debridement and surgical approach, fails in about fifteen to twenty percent of treated individuals, the so-called refractory patients."

The bacteria that form, live, and grow in plaque have to be removed. When certain species of these bacteria grow into large numbers, gingivitis, then gum disease set in. Gingivitis is merely the very beginning stage of gum disease.

Unfortunately, society has accepted the concept of the slowly receding gum line. This acceptance is evident in the phrase, "growing long in the tooth," which is occasionally heard even today. For those who wish to maintain a youthful appearance, receding gum tissue is one more battlefront in that particular war.

Gum disease is a serious condition; it can lead to tooth loss. However, an increasing number of studies are pointing to the contribution of gum disease to cardiovascular problems. Plaque is constantly accumulating on everyone's teeth. There is no person who does not accumulate plaque on his/her teeth and gums. This plaque gives bacteria a chance to grow.

What this means is that virtually all of us are susceptible to gum disease. I have read that about two percent of the population is apparently immune to gum disease. Sadly, the rest of us do not share the genes or the other factors that may have caused such a superior situation.

This indicates that ninety-eight percent of us need to be concerned about this potential killer, if not for the sake of preventing the loss of our teeth, then perhaps for the sake of reducing the risk of cardiovascular disease. I would prefer to keep my own teeth and not have to hassle with dentures or implants. Neither absolves you of taking care of your gums, anyway. You would still have to continue to maintain their health.

Statistics speak of gum disease occurring prevalently in individuals over thirty-five years of age. However, consider that if gum disease is a chronically progressing problem, then it must begin at a much younger age. It is just that the results are not obvious until the receded gum line becomes more noticeable.

Therefore, whatever a person's age, one needs to start thinking about what to do to prevent gum disease or stop the progression if it has already begun. Finally, though caring for the teeth and gums via brushing and flossing are very helpful, they cannot be considered enough to always stop gum disease in all people based on the large number of the adult population that currently displays some form of gum disease.

If brushing and flossing your teeth is not enough to prevent gum disease, then perhaps there are other tools that can help. If so, what else do you need to do to fight against or prevent gum disease?

In short, we must be very diligent no matter where we are in our current state of gum health. If you have not seen any signs of gingivitis yet, you should want to work on preventing future problems. If you have seen those signs, then it is time to work on halting the progression of the disease now, before it takes away any more of your gum tissue or causes the loss of any teeth. Since it is generally believed that eroded gum tissue will not regenerate, or will only do so to a limited extent, the time to start preventing or controlling an existing case of gum disease is precisely now.

This article is for information purposes only and is not meant to suggest treatment, prevention, or diagnosis of any oral health condition. If you have or think you might have an oral health problem, you should contact your dentist for diagnosis and treatment right away.

David Snape is the author of the book, *What You Should Know about Gum Disease*. You can find Dave and ask questions about gum disease or other health, fitness, or wellness topics at: http://whatyoushouldknowaboutgumdisease.com. David practices the gentle but powerful exercises of Falun Gong. You can read about, and watch video instructions for, these exercises at http://www.FalunDafa.org.

Loose Teeth

Gum disease can cause damage to the underlying bone structure that supports your gums and holds your teeth in place. This bone and tissue is relatively vulnerable and can be damaged by the effects of bacterial infection.

Some have the notion that only people in their thirties and forties develop gum disease. Let's think about that for a minute. Where did that gum disease come from? Could it have developed over the last ten, twenty, or thirty years? Gingivitis is the beginning stage of gum disease and has been detected in people of all ages.

When a bacterial infection occurs under the gum line, the supporting structure is attacked by the by-products secreted from the bacteria. Once this structure is eroded, you might also notice that the gums have receded. Again, this did not happen overnight.

One key to avoiding gum disease is to realize that odds are fairly high you will develop it if you do not already have it. By creating good habits while in your teens or twenties, you can prevent the onset of gum disease later in life. You will be able to keep your teeth when others lose theirs.

Once the supporting bone structure is compromised, the teeth become loose, depending on how bad the damage is. At some point, the supporting structure will not be strong enough to support the tooth at all and then it is over. The tooth is lost.

As an adult, there is no replacement tooth unless you count dentures or implants. Gum disease is the number one cause of tooth loss. Every person on the planet, except for the rare two percent who are heavily gum disease resistant, needs to worry about this problem. Make a plan to prevent or combat it and execute that plan on a daily basis.

Starting early is the key to prevention. However, if you failed to start early, you can begin to take steps to prevent your situation from becoming worse. If you fail to take any action, there are still options. However, you will not necessarily like those options.

I remember that an older man at a recent gathering said, "There is no substitute for your own teeth." Implants or dentures are poor substitutes for the real thing. I do not believe most people are too lazy to take care of their teeth. Instead, I believe they do not understand what will happen if they don't—or lack the knowledge necessary to do an adequate job. After all, the only advice most people get is to "brush and floss" and maybe, "use mouthwash." How many people understand that most of the adult population is afflicted by some stage of gum disease? Most go through their daily lives oblivious to what is happening just inside their own mouths.

Some people make a distinction between gingivitis and gum disease. One is just the beginning of the other. If you are in your twenties or

225

teens and have been told you have gingivitis, now is the time to become diligent about oral care. Today's gingivitis can develop into tomorrow's periodontal disease. It is just a matter of degree.

Unfortunately, the public is woefully ignorant of gum disease, what it is, and what it can do to you as an individual. Again, gum disease is the number one cause of tooth loss. A popoular clinic's website quips that perhaps up to eighty percent of the adult population in America has gum disease. Many Americans are fanatical about taking care of their smiles. Yet so many still develop this disease.

You owe it to yourself to find out everything you can to prevent gum disease, or fight it once you become aware of it. Ask your dentist about the health of your gums every time you go for a checkup. If you have bleeding during your normal cleaning, you should be aware this is not normal. Even if you bleed a little bit, it could very well indicate you have gingivitis or gum disease. The gums are not sore to the touch in a healthy situation. Healthy gums should not feel painful when being probed or prodded.

In addition to the health of your gums, the overall health of your body should also be considered. It is arguably the most important aspect of your life. If you have or think you might have gum disease, contact your dentist for diagnosis, advice, and treatment.

David Snape is the author of the book, What You Should Know about Gum Disease. You can find Dave and ask questions about gum disease or other health, fitness, or wellness topics at:
http://whatyoushouldknowaboutgumdisease.com.

Dental Plaque and Gum Disease
Plaque is a biofilm that can start to reform about 30 minutes after

removing it. Inside the plaque, bacteria find a nice place to hide and begin to multiply rapidly. The plaque provides optimal conditions for bacterial proliferation.

The first type of bacteria that forms within the plaque is the gram-positive bacteria. They are not deemed to be the bacteria responsible for gum disease. It is the second type, the gram-negative bacteria, that is believed to cause gum disease. The gram-negative bacteria begin to inhabit and multiply in the plaque about two days after plaque forms. These gram-negative bacteria produce an acid waste product that is detrimental to both tooth enamel and gum tissue.

This is why flossing is so vitally important. It is an efficient mechanical way to remove plaque from between and around the teeth.

If you floss daily, it should help to prevent or fight gum disease. However, some dental professionals have a different recommendation. Regardless of what you read here, you should only follow the directions of your dentist, doctor, or periodontist.

There are still questions to consider. Are you really getting all of the plaque off when you floss? Are you missing any? Do you miss the same spots all of the time?

If you miss the same spots all of the time, then you are not getting rid of the plaque in that area at all. It is able to facilitate the rapid growth and provide a breeding ground for the harmful bacteria that causes gum disease. This is another reason why professional care is so important. Your hygienist can help you to discover the spots you are missing on a regular basis.

Since so many people have gum disease, it seems unlikely that regular brushing and flossing, regardless of the reason, is enough to stop gum disease. Perhaps people do not floss thoroughly enough. Perhaps, they do not floss long enough. Whatever the reason, the statistics tell us that a lot of people are walking around with some form of gum disease.

The question becomes, what does work to rid oneself of gum disease? I was told by a periodontist that a study conducted in Scandinavia indicated that getting a professional cleaning once every two months cleared up a lot of problems associated with gum disease.

Unfortunately, most insurance companies will not or do not recognize this as the standard of care that should be maintained. I was also told that the once-every-six-month model of professional cleaning was originally intended to fight dental cavities and not gum disease. Gum disease is a different ball game that requires more frequent professional cleaning as well as good home care.

I was told that I had gum disease, and that I needed a root scaling and planing treatment. I declined and bought a special device called a Hydro Floss and used it daily. When I went in for my next dental checkup I was told that I did not need that scaling and root planing treatment any longer.

My gums do not bleed upon brushing and flossing any longer. If you have gums that bleed while brushing or flossing, that is often a sign of gum disease. No one ever told me that. In fact, I never knew it until I started researching gum disease. Be aware that if you have any bleeding while brushing or flossing, you possibly have gum disease. Most people are not aware of this basic fact. As in my case, they often think bleeding is normal.

This article just provides basic information that may or may not be deemed correct by dental professionals or other experts. If you have or think you have gum disease, you should visit your dentist for diagnosis, treatment, and prevention advice.

David Snape is the author of the book, *What You Should Know about Gum Disease*. You can find Dave and ask questions about gum disease or other health, fitness, or wellness topics at: http://whatyoushouldknowaboutgumdisease.com.

The FYI on Gum Disease

Do you wonder about the health of your gums? Do your gums appear red, puffy, or swollen? Do you experience bleeding when brushing, flossing, or visiting the dentist's office? Have you grown "long in the tooth?" Have you lost any teeth due to gum disease? Know anyone else who has?

Eighty percent of American adults suffer from some form of gum disease according to the Mayo Clinic's website. The question that begs to be answered is, why? Eighty percent? That is quite a high number. No one ever talks about gum disease, which leads me to believe that out of that eighty percent, few realize they suffer from it. Eighty percent equates to eight out of ten people.

That means most of the people you know, possibly including yourself, suffer from some form of gum disease. Many people probably do not know they have gum disease. They will in the future, though, because eventually their dentist will tell them that they need a scaling and root planing, surgery, or periodontal work done, or they will lose a tooth. Then they will suddenly become aware of what gum disease can do!

The Surgeon General once described oral and dental disease as a silent epidemic. Studies continue to surface that suggest gum disease could be a precursor to larger problems such as heart disease. Gum disease can be a route by which bacteria and other pathogens enter the body. Having gum disease means that you have left a door open to infection.

Despite all of this, few people talk about gum disease and even fewer are doing anything about it. I can foresee a day when people will pay particular attention to their oral health, because it will become common knowledge of just how serious the situation with our gum tissue is. At least, I hope it enters the mainstream awareness soon. People need to know about it.

Unfortunately, many people will lose precious gum tissue before they even realize that they have this disease, or before their dentist mentions it to them. That is why the time is precisely now to start working on this, regardless of what stage of oral health you are at. Protecting your gum tissue is protecting your overall health if all the suspected links to other disease are real.

If you are anything like me, you went on for quite some time thinking it did not matter if your gums bled a little during brushing or flossing. Nothing is further from the truth. If you experience any bleeding at all while brushing and flossing, that is probably indicating an abnormal and possibly already diseased condition. Check with your dentist for diagnosis, advice, and treatment.

Since as many as eighty percent of adult Americans suffer from this disease, it is reasonable to suspect that the preventive measures of brushing and flossing that we were all taught are not adequate to prevent or stop gum disease. If you are like me, you will one day discover that you have suffered from this disease and have lost bone and tissue as result, unknowingly and without much fanfare.

I was determined not to lose any teeth to this villain and I researched and tested a number of tools that I could use to arrest the progress of gum disease and keep it away. I wrote the book, *What You Should Know about Gum Disease* as a result.

This article is for informational purposes only. Check with your dentist if you have or think you might have gum disease for advice, diagnosis and treatment.

David Snape is the author of the book, *What You Should Know about Gum Disease.* You can find Dave and ask questions about gum disease or other health, fitness, or wellness topics at:

http://whatyoushouldknowaboutgumdisease.com.

Long in the Tooth?
Few things are as discouraging as seeing your gums recede. There is a difference between healthy gums and non-healthy gums. Getting "long in the tooth" is not necessarily something that automatically has to happen with age. It is largely a function or by-product of gum disease. However, rough brushing habits can also be a problem.

Many official sources say that poor oral hygiene is the cause of gum disease. I sometimes wonder if they are not just echoing each other because no one adequately explains what poor oral hygiene is. Consider that as many as seventy-five or eighty percent of the adult population may be afflicted with gum disease. If professionals are adequately explaining good oral hygiene, should the numbers be so high?

One has to wonder about two things: Is poor oral hygiene the cause of gum disease? If so, what is good oral hygiene? I used to go to a dentist every six months to get my teeth cleaned. When it comes to explaining oral hygiene, I only heard the mantra about brushing, flossing, and using mouthwash. Those are the things I have always done. Yet, I still developed gum disease.

I am pretty particular about brushing and flossing and always have been. However, I still developed this disease. When I was told that I could lose my teeth and that they wanted to do special treatments on me, I began to ponder these questions and more.

Theories about gum disease and talk about its prevalence abound. Universally, virtually everyone agrees that plaque and tartar buildup (a.k.a. calculus) are the cause of gum disease. These substances harbor anaerobic bacteria.

Therefore, the next question becomes: How can I prevent plaque buildup? Once again, the answer generally returns to brushing and flossing.

This is the circle that the puzzle of gum disease revolves within. I do not know that what is taught about brushing and flossing by the dentists I have visited over the years is adequate.

For me personally, I used to floss with a basic up and down motion. I did that between each of my teeth and then I was finished. However, recently I began using both an up and down and back and forth motion. This revealed sore spots in my gums that I had not been able to find before. You should still learn about proper flossing techniques from your dentist's office.

If your gums bleed during brushing or flossing, there is a good chance you have gum disease. You will need your dentist to confirm that for you and rule out any other problems. However, bleeding gums are usually a symptom of gum disease.

I spent some time doing a little research and gained a lot of experience trying out different things that could improve the health of my gums without the need to give up the foods and snacks that I enjoy. In order to share this information with others, I wrote: *What You Should Know about Gum Disease.*

If you have or think you might have gingivitis, gum disease, or any other oral health problem, visit your dentist for diagnosis and treatment.

David Snape is the author of the book, *What You Should Know about Gum Disease.* You can find Dave and ask questions about gum disease or other health, fitness, or wellness topics at: http://whatyoushouldknowaboutgumdisease.com.

Why is Gum Disease so Prevalent?

With our incredibly busy lifestyles, it is virtually impossible to take into account everything that either needs to be done or should be done on a daily basis. Those things that require less immediate action in the present, such as retirement planning and gingivitis, tend to receive less attention from us.

In addition, gum disease is something most people do not think about until it becomes obvious they have it. Therefore, they do not become aware that their oral care routine is not adequate until gum recession, loose teeth, or other problems show up. Unfortunately, once gum disease has gotten a foothold, it is harder to get rid of it. An ounce of prevention is worth more than a pound of cure in the case of gum disease.

There can be other factors that contribute to the problem, as well. If you grind your teeth, this excessive force can put tremendous mechanical pressure on the supporting structure of your gums and teeth and weaken that structure. This makes it easier for gum disease to progress.

If you have crooked teeth, the plaque that forms a nice home for bacteria finds places to exist that your daily care routine might not reach very well. Straight teeth are important for more reasons than just having a pretty smile. Unfortunately, I myself have suffered from gum disease, and it is hard to arrest the progress in places where the teeth are not straight. It is relatively easier to get to the places of my mouth where the teeth are not crowded together.

Flossing is very important, but I have found that flossing is not enough to prevent plaque buildup and calculus formation on my teeth and near my gums. It remains a mystery to me. However, I believe I am not alone in this. I have read stories of others who have taken good care of their teeth conscientiously with regular brushing and flossing, yet could not stop the accumulation of plaque.

I have spent a great deal of time to find tools that would help me fight gum disease and prevent its progress. Some tools have more value than others do.

Unfortunately, if the information provided by our professionals was adequate to prevent gum disease, then the statistics would not be so horrendous. Most quip that as many as seventy-five percent of people over thirty-five have some sort of gum disease. The Mayo Clinic website said that eighty percent of adult Americans are afflicted in some way. Whichever of the many statements out there are most accurate does not matter—it's a lot of people! This should not be the case.

With this prevalence of gum disease, not much needs to be said. You can ponder for yourself whether regular brushing and flossing are enough to prevent this problem. If you have or think you might have gum disease, be sure to visit your periodontist for advice, diagnosis, and treatment.

David Snape is the author of the book, *What You Should Know about Gum Disease.* You can find Dave and ask questions about gum disease or other health, fitness, or wellness topics at: http://whatyoushouldknowaboutgumdisease.com.

Anti-Aging and Your Gums

Have you ever considered how your gums affect your apparent state of youth? Ever hear the phrase, "growing long in the tooth?" This refers directly to recession of the gums. The look of a smile is something that people usually consider when assessing age.

If you are youthful, your gum tissue might not have had enough time to recede under the influence of infecting bacteria. However, twenty years later, plenty of time has gone by for gum disease to have slowly done its damage. Since that damage often accumulates over time, you probably will not notice it until you approach middle age. Yet many people already have gum disease at an even earlier age. The visible damage becomes evident later.

Fortunately you can prevent gum disease. Or, if you have already noticed your gum line receding, you can slow or stop its progression. Gum recession is most often a byproduct of chronic gum disease. Over time, the health of the gum tissue is compromised by the buildup of plaque and tartar near and under the gum line. When this happens, the gums become irritated and they begin to separate from the tooth. Over time, the health of the underlying bone structure begins to disintegrate as a result of bacterial infection. Then, the gums recede further because there is no longer enough bone to hold them up. In addition, they continue to be attacked by toxins that bacteria produce. By working to keep your gums healthy you can avoid the "long in the tooth" appearance.

Our mouths are inherently dirty places. Every time we eat food, the teeth grind and rend our meal into smaller pieces. Most of those pieces get swallowed for further processing to provide calories and nutrients to the body. A smaller percentage of those food particles are mashed around and end up resting on or near our gum tissue. These particles sit there until the next time you rinse, brush, and floss.

The bacteria that are naturally present in our mouth feast on this food, too, especially on sugars. In addition, if you have eaten food that decreases the pH of the mouth or dries it (as in the case of alcohol), you will find that the environment becomes favorable for the bacteria, which are able to multiply more rapidly.

Keeping your gum tissue healthy requires a little bit more than just brushing and flossing. Since eighty percent of America's adult population may have some form of gum disease, according to the Mayo Clinic's estimate, there is a good chance that you or someone you love has this disease. It is quiet and lurks in the background of your life, scarcely noticeable, until one day you start to see the difference show up in your smile.

Once the gum tissue has eroded, you will probably need to have special treatments and possibly surgery to attempt to restore it. Why not avoid all that hassle and expense in the first place via prevention?

My dentist told me I had gum disease. They wanted to do what is called a scaling and root planing on my teeth. This involves scraping along the root of the tooth to remove tartar buildup. I declined, as that sounded both costly and painful. I also read that in many cases such a treatment has to be repeated. In addition, I know someone who had it done and she was not happy with the results.

Upon searching for an alternative that I could apply at home without a lot of cost or hassle, I stumbled across the right combination of tools to help me combat gum disease. As a result, the hygienist told me that I no longer needed a scaling and root planing the next time I visited. The last time I went, there was no bleeding on probing to indicate gum disease.

Our smiles can give away our age. Protecting our gums by preventing gingivitis and gum disease can help us maintain a more youthful appearance. However, if you have gum disease or think you might, visit a dentist for diagnosis and treatment.

David Snape is the author of the book, *What You Should Know about Gum Disease.* You can find Dave and ask questions about gum disease or other health, fitness, or wellness topics at: http://whatyoushouldknowaboutgumdisease.com.

Why Gum Disease?
Gum disease is both an interesting and terrible phenomenon. The prevalence of gum disease can really be blamed on the "out of sight, out of mind" blind spot that human beings have. Preparing and planning are not one of our strong suits as a species. We lack the ability to foresee very far or very much into the future.

In addition, our days are filled with many things to keep us busy. We simply cannot maintain focus on every aspect of every detail that might affect us in the future.

Hence, we have this problem with gum disease. You often hear that gum disease afflicts people in their mid-thirties and above. Actually, it has been found in children as young as six years old. Gum disease does not just show up magically at the age of thirty-five. No, it has been present for quite some time. It just becomes evident for most people in their thirties. However, it can become evident at any age—it is a myth to think it only affects people over thirty. That is simply when many people start to take notice of the damage that has been accumulating all along.

When tissue is younger, the evidence of the disease is not apparent when you look in the mirror. Yet it is precisely this time when you have to start worrying about gum disease; if we do not work on preventing its progression at the time when it is not visible, there will not be as much wiggle room when it does become evident.

Generally, it is believed that receded gum tissue will not regenerate. Therefore, once you become "long in the tooth," there are less options available. You can possibly get a periodontist to do some expensive, time-consuming and painful work to get your receded gum line back. The results will probably not be what you hoped for. Why let it get there in the first place?

Why let it get there in the first place?
Tartar buildup is the big issue. Plaque forms so fast and so readily that it is difficult to keep it off. You have to brush and floss daily. Yet, over time, brushing and flossing alone may not be enough to prevent gum disease for many people.

Another modern invention that has helped many people control the progression of gum disease is the oral irrigator. I personally like to use the Hydro Floss. It is powerful and employs something that other irrigators do not: hydromagnetics.

You can find information on a study that indicates the potential effectiveness of the Hydro Floss at:

http://tobeinformed.com/228/.

Since the Mayo Clinic website suggests that about eighty percent of adult Americans are afflicted with gum disease, it is reasonable to assume that regular brushing and flossing are not enough. Therefore, oral irrigation could be a helpful addition to your normal daily oral hygiene regimen.

If you have or think you have a dental health problem, including gum disease, visit your dentist for diagnosis and treatment. This article is for entertainment and information purposes only and is not meant to advise in any way.

David Snape is the author of the book, *What You Should Know about Gum Disease*. You can find Dave and ask questions about gum disease or other health, fitness, or wellness topics at:

http://whatyoushouldknowaboutgumdisease.com.

Gum Disease and a Person's Future
I see them frequently. They have partial or full plates or implants, which are not their original teeth. I do not know about you, but I would like to keep my original teeth for a lifetime.

According to a popular clinic's website, eighty percent of adult Americans suffer form gum disease. In case you have not guessed by now, this is exactly what is responsible for the tooth loss of the majority of our adult population.

Unfortunately, gum disease is something that starts early and takes its toll silently, over several decades. Then one day, you get surprised with the news that you are going to need your teeth pulled or that you have gum disease. This scenario can often be avoided.

I do not know if this has happened to you or will happen to you, but my hygienist one day shocked me with the news that she wanted me to sign a paper saying it was not her fault if I lost my teeth!

I have been going to the same dentist for years, and was never told what I need to do to prevent this disease from getting worse, nor how important it was to do so. Yet, suddenly she wanted me to sign something saying she and the dentist were not responsible.

Unfortunately, if flossing and brushing alone were always the answer, the eighty percent statistic would not be so high. I have seen a similar stat on the National Institute of Health's site, as well. I brush more gently now because my investigation and experience has taught me that it is not necessary to brush hard. Of course, flossing is also very important and should be done.

By far the most important device I have and that I use every day, often more than once per day, is the Hydro Floss:

http://whatyoushouldknowaboutgumdisease.com.

That is the first device I found that actually stopped my gums from bleeding during brushing, flossing, and at the dentist's office. This was the first hurdle on the road to recovery. However, for me the battle might never be over. I have lost some of my gum tissue and I really need to be diligent to prevent the return of gum disease. I cannot afford to lose any more gum tissue if I want to keep my teeth for the rest of my life.

If your gum disease has not progressed very far yet, get to work on better prevention now. If it has progressed, then you need to work even harder to stop it and prevent it from coming back and progressing further.

This is something that almost every human being needs to think about. There is only about two percent of the population that is immune to gum disease; just two percent. That means ninety-eight percent of us can or will get it.

In any case, it is best to learn everything you can now. Talk to your dentist about the Hydro Floss and see if it is right for you. If you have or think you might have gum disease or any other health problem, visit your periodontist or dentist for advice, diagnosis, and treatment. The FDA has not evaluated statements about any products mentioned.

David Snape is the author of the book, *What You Should Know about Gum Disease*. You can find Dave and ask questions about gum disease or other health, fitness, or wellness topics at:

http://whatyoushouldknowaboutgumdisease.com.

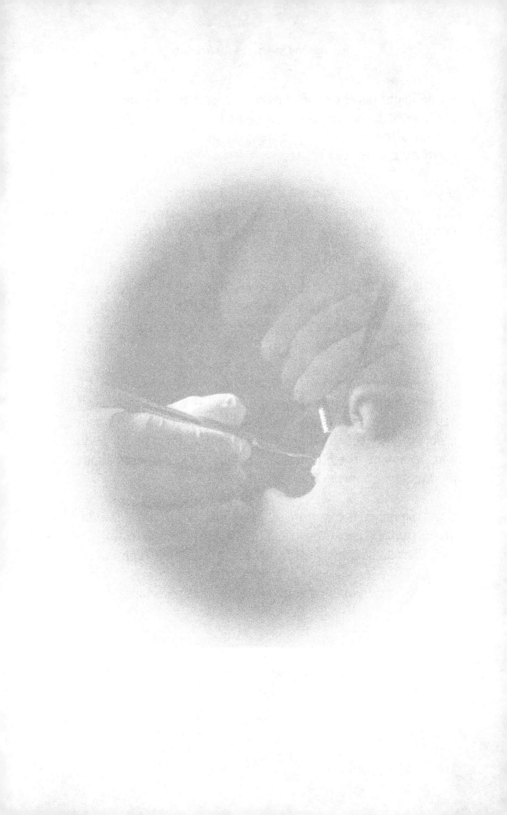

About The Author

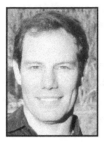 David Snape grew up in New Jersey, not far from the Atlantic Ocean.

He joined the Navy at eighteen and worked as an aviation electronics technician. He worked in many areas of the country and was eventually assigned to a duty station in Hawaii.

Upon leaving the military, he started preparing for a career in health.

Due to a number of factors and growing disillusionment with his chosen profession and future colleagues, he left professional training early, never to return.

He soon found himself working in toxicology, then information technology. All the while, he never lost his passion for health and wellness information, and created the ToBeInformed website as an outlet for those interests.

Despite all his training and background, he was caught totally off guard by gum disease and the damage it could cause. Once he made this discovery, he knew that others should be informed and wrote the book, *What You Should Know About Gum Disease*.

Ever since high school, David has been concerned about injustice, human rights, and the sufferings of others. He was shocked to learn of the brutal persecution of Falun Dafa, the meditation practice he eventually settled upon after much soul-searching.

In February 2002, he traveled to China to protest these massive human rights violations—along with western practitioners of Falun Gong from many different countries. The communist rulers of China met their message of Truth, Compassion, Tolerance, and peaceful, non-violent protest with contempt, and they were all deported from the country.

While many others benefit from this ancient qigong practice around the world, the persecution of Falun Gong is ongoing in China. David continues to work behind the scenes to help raise awareness, with the eventual goal of ending the persecution of Falun Gong in China.